Natural Healing Foods Encyclopedia

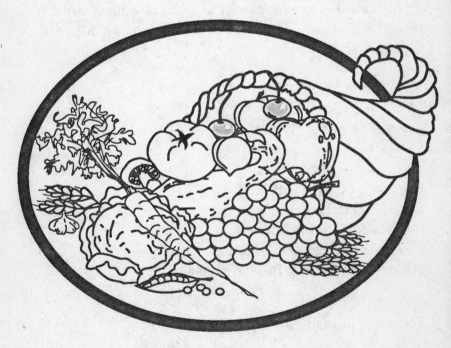

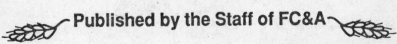 Published by the Staff of FC&A

FC&A Publishing
103 Clover Green
Peachtree City, GA 30269

Publisher: FC&A Publishing
Editor: Cal Beverly
Production: Carol Parrott
Cover Design: Deberah Williams
Printed and bound by Banta Company

Second printing February 1992

ISBN 0-915099-37-3

Contents

How to Cope
with Cholesterol 33

Notice to the reader

Changing your diet to achieve optimum healthiness, to lose or gain weight and to derive maximum disease prevention are serious personal decisions. Such decisions should be discussed thoroughly in advance with your doctor or healthcare provider.

Some people have medical conditions that make a change in their diets inadvisable or even dangerous. Before going on any new diet, you should discuss your options and any potential hazards with your doctor.

The authors, editors and publishers have been diligent in attempting to provide you with accurate information in this book. However, with the rapid advances in nutrition research and medical science, we recommend that you contact your own physician before taking or discontinuing any foods or beverages, nutrients, medicines or drugs and before treating yourself in any way.

This publication does not constitute medical practice or advice. Its only intent is to provide you, the consumer, with easy-to-understand information.

May God be with you as you strive for a healthy life!

"Your body, you know, is the temple of the Holy Spirit, who is in you since you received Him from God You are not your own property. You have been bought and paid for. This is why you should use your body for the glory of God."

— 1 Corinthians 6:19–20.

CHAPTER 1

Introduction

An introduction to healing foods

Not all medicine is manufactured, and not all cures come out of a pill bottle.

That's the lesson being re-learned today by many health-care professionals, medical students and consumers.

The things we eat and drink promote far-reaching effects in our bodies, for good and for ill. In recent years, we have come to a new understanding of what "nourishment" really means.

Every day, medical researchers document new evidences of the healing properties available in many foods. And new research points out the disadvantages of consuming some of the foods and beverages we may have come to enjoy and depend on.

In this book, we bring together some of that research to help you find your way through a maze of nutritional opinions.

In the first section, we consider the overall question — What is a healthy diet?

CHAPTER 2

Good Nutrition

Build a healthy diet foundation

You might think it's "too late" to change your eating habits, but that's far from true. You can bet that changing your eating habits today will go a long way toward promoting good health tomorrow, regardless of your age.

Especially for people over age 50, more health problems are caused by poor nutrition and lack of exercise than by aging alone, indicates a report in *Geriatrics* (44,6:57). Many older people fail to get even the official recommended daily allowances of vitamins and minerals necessary for good health.

For example, of those over age 60, more than half the men and more than seven out of every 10 women don't get enough folic acid (a B-vitamin) and vitamin B6, according to the *Geriatrics* report.

In that same age group, about five of every 10 men and six of every 10 women fall short of getting enough vitamin D.

Smaller percentages in that age group have problems

getting enough zinc, calcium, vitamin B12 and vitamin A.

There are many reasons. First, many people don't know what the recommended daily allowances are. Secondly, they don't know what foods to eat or drink to meet the requirements. And in a few cases, aging digestive systems don't process certain vitamins and minerals as well as in younger years.

Although researchers are still studying the particular nutritional needs of older Americans, moderation seems to be the key to good health. Maintain a low-salt, low-fat, well-balanced diet by eating a variety of fruits, vegetables, whole grains and lean meats. Limit your intake of alcohol, and talk to your physician about an exercise program. Regular exercise will help you keep up a healthy appetite.

The foods you eat — and how much you eat — have a big impact on your risk of developing certain diseases, especially heart disease, according to a report in *The American Journal of Clinical Nutrition* (49,5:995).

"Diet, through caloric, salt, alcohol, and fat intake, plays a fundamental role in the development of cardiovascular disease," the report says. Excess amounts of meat, eggs, animal protein and animal fat are related to heart disease, and excess salt and alcohol are related to hypertension. Obesity has been linked with stroke, liver and heart diseases, and problems during surgery.

Vitamins alone won't keep you healthy, and excess doses can be toxic. Therefore, discuss with your doctor your plans for taking vitamin and mineral supplements.

"By taking a vitamin pill, people think they are maintaining their health and are distracted from controlling the factors that will have the most impact on their health—total fat, calories and cholesterol," says a report in *Archives of Internal Medicine* (149,6:1254).

Take these good-nutrition tips from nutritionist Nancy Clark, who outlines a "foundation diet" in *Senior Patient* (1,5:95). She encourages you to eat more of these good foods:

Dairy Products — Even if you're watching cholesterol, don't eliminate dairy foods entirely, she advises. Choose non-fat (rather than low-fat) products, which have all the vitamins and minerals you need without the fat. You should have three servings of dairy products each day.
Try a cup of non-fat yogurt with fruit with lunch or add powered milk to mashed potatoes. A hefty scoop of cottage cheese has only 130 milligrams of calcium but a whopping 20 grams of protein (equivalent to a quarter-pound hamburger before it's cooked).

Fruits — Orange and grapefruit juices are more nutritious than other fruit juices, such as apple, grape and cranberry— and they're lower in calories, too. A six-ounce glass of orange juice will provide your daily requirement of vitamin C. But eating the whole fruit is better than drinking a glass of juice, according to the nutritionist.
Bananas are potassium-rich and have only about 100 calories—a good afternoon snack. Spread peanut butter on top for extra protein.

Vegetables—Choose dark, colorful vegetables—romaine

lettuce, spinach, green peppers, broccoli and carrots. One carrot—whether cooked or grated into a salad—will also provide the recommended daily allowance of vitamin A or its equivalent in beta carotene, the report says. Celery, cucumbers, onions and radishes have a greater "crunch factor" but are not as nutritious.

Another way to get your RDA of vitamin C is to eat "one stalk of cooked broccoli, half a green pepper, two medium tomatoes or a spinach salad." Avoid canned or processed tomatoes, which are high in sodium. Tomato juice and sauce are fine and "are as nutritious as fresh tomatoes." Winter squash is high in vitamin A and potassium.

Potatoes are nutrient-rich (potassium, fiber and vitamin C), can be prepared many ways and are better for you than rice or noodles. Potatoes are not fattening; what you put on them is. Avoid butter, sour cream and gravies. Try instead a baked potato with a butter substitute or a little skim milk and "mash" the potato.

Don't overcook vegetables. They will retain more nutrients if they're microwaved or steamed rather than boiled.

Starches — Generally, darker breads are more nutritious than refined white breads. Whole-wheat, bran and rye breads are fiber-rich. Try a slice with a thin spread of peanut butter. Freeze bread to keep it fresh; it takes only a few minutes for slices to thaw.

Bran cereals are good sources of fiber and iron and help lower cholesterol. "Look for the words 'enriched' or 'fortified' on the labels," the nutritionist suggests. To get a healthy start in the morning, try bran cereal with skim milk, a banana and a glass of orange juice.

Meat and Fish — Nutritionists recommend two weekly servings of fish, which keep your heart healthy and is easy to prepare. "Put the fish in a shallow pan, add a little water, cover and cook over medium heat for about five minutes until it flakes easily when pierced with a fork," Nancy Clark says.
Choose extra-lean ground beef and turkey — good sources of protein, vitamins, iron and zinc. Limit beef to three four-ounce servings a week. Commercially prepared turkey usually has more fat and calories than turkey prepared at home.

Treats — "Fig newtons, raisin squares, animal crackers and gingersnaps are acceptable treats because they're lower in saturated fats than most desserts and offer slightly more nutritional value than chocolate chip cookies," she says in the report.

RDA for those over 50

The following tables give the official Recommended Dietary Allowances for vitamins and minerals in amounts considered necessary for people over age 50.
The tables contain two measurement categories — (1) those vitamins and minerals that are needed in milligram amounts; and (2) those needed in much smaller microgram amounts. Scientists usually measure nutrients in units called

milligrams and micrograms. A milligram is one-thousandth of a gram. A microgram is one-thousandth of a milligram, or one-millionth of a gram. For comparison, it takes more than 28 grams to equal one ounce, and there are 16 ounces in one pound.

	Vitamins	
	Males	Females
Vitamin A	1,000 micrograms	800 micrograms
Vitamin D	5 micrograms	5 micrograms
Vitamin E	10 milligrams	8 milligrams
Vitamin C	60 milligrams	60 milligrams
Folacin (Folic Acid)	200 micrograms	180 micrograms
Niacin	15 milligrams	13 milligrams
Riboflavin	1.4 milligrams	1.2 milligrams
Thiamine	1.2 milligrams	1 milligram
Vitamin B6	2 milligrams	1.6 milligrams
Vitamin B12	2 micrograms	2 micrograms
Vitamin K	80 micrograms	65 micrograms
	Minerals	
	Males	Females
Calcium	800 milligrams	800 milligrams
Phosphorous	800 milligrams	800 milligrams
Iodine	150 micrograms	150 micrograms
Iron	10 milligrams	10 milligrams
Magnesium	350 milligrams	280 milligrams
Selenium	70 micrograms	55 micrograms
Zinc	15 milligrams	12 milligrams

The chart is based on the National Research Council's publication, *Recommended Dietary Allowances—10th Edition* (National Academy Press, Washington, D.C., 1989).

People on medications or on special, restricted diets should check with their doctors before using the information above. Certain nutrients — like selenium — are dangerous in amounts only slightly above the recommended range. Check with your doctor before taking any vitamin or mineral supplements.

All about fresh vegetables and how to cook them

Just about every day, you are told to eat plain vegetables. The reason is simple: vegetables are generally high in vitamins and fiber.

Additional soluble fiber, protein and vitamins B and E may be added to vegetables by including oat bran. Vegetables with a distinct texture — such as broccoli — may simply be sprinkled with oat bran before serving. Vegetables that are more smooth in texture often taste good when soaked in a marinade prepared with a small amount of oat bran.

Vegetables are one type of food that will actually help your weight-reduction diet. Most have only 20 to 50 calories per cup. Plus their bulk helps you feel full, making more fattening foods less tempting.

One trick practiced by many dieters is to keep fresh

carrot and celery sticks cut up in the refrigerator at all times. They provide a satisfying, crunchy snack while causing virtually no damage to the waistline.

Unfortunately, many of us grew up eating canned vegetables that were loaded down with salt and fat when cooked. To take advantage of all the nutrition in vegetables:

- Choose fresh vegetables over ones that have been processed and packaged. With a little practice they are as easy to prepare as canned ones and have the advantage of not having been processed to death. Your second choice should be frozen vegetables.
- Learn to ask questions in the produce section of the supermarket. Find out which vegetables were picked ripe. Some lose a major portion of the nutritive value when picked unripe and then stored before being offered for sale. Also, avoid obviously bruised or wilted vegetables.
- Unfortunately, vegetables lose nutrients as they wait to be eaten — and many lose some of their flavor. Plan to eat fresh vegetables as soon as possible. Do not buy more fresh vegetables then may be eaten within three or four days. Always store fresh produce in your refrigerator's crisper or in moisture-proof bags.
- Not all vegetables are compatible in storage. Apples make carrots bitter and onions speed up spoilage in potatoes.
- Cut the leaves off of carrots and other root vegetables before storing. Vitamins continue to leave the root and travel up into the leaves even after being pulled from the ground.
- Always carefully wash vegetables before using, but avoid

leaving them in water for any length of time.

Baking for health

Using coarse flour for routine baking may lower your risk of getting high blood pressure, hardening of the arteries, gallstones, obesity and diseases of the colon, even colon cancer, a new report says.

That's the suggestion from three doctors at the Bristol Royal Infirmary in England, as reported in *British Medical Journal* (298,6688:1616).

Part of the healthful effect of coarsely ground flour may be because it escapes complete digestion in the stomach and upper intestines, the doctors say.

"Overefficient digestion of starch" may give rise to excess levels of insulin in the blood and to problems with the colon, the lower end of the digestive tract, the report suggests.

Some doctors think that some cases of high blood pressure may be triggered by problems with insulin levels.

Undigested coarse flour also could beneficially affect the colon like rough dietary fiber, the doctors say.

For those reasons, they tested the theory on 20 patients who either suffered from non-insulin-dependent diabetes or had undergone colon surgery to treat ulcerative colitis.

"In both groups, the meal containing bread made from coarse flour resulted in lower plasma glucose and insulin concentrations than that containing bread made from fine flour," the report says.

"Thus the risk of some colonic diseases, including cancer, might be reduced if coarse flour was eaten regularly and combined with other less completely digested starchy foods," the doctors conclude.

The researchers also suggest that diabetics may achieve better control of blood sugar levels by eating breads baked from coarse flour.

Here's how the doctors measure whether flour is coarse: nearly half the flour will not pass through a sieve with holes one millimeter wide, and at least 80 percent of the flour won't pass through holes of 140 micrometers diameter.

What not to add

Avoid the temptation to toss your vegetables in a pan of water with salt and fatback. Not only will this add unhealthy fat and sodium to your diet, it subtracts vitamins and minerals.

Your best choices for cooking vegetables are the microwave and a steamer. Most kitchen supply stores carry expandable steamers which may be placed in the bottom of any sized pot with a tight-fitting lid. Be aware that some vegetables cook best by using a combination of boiling and steaming. This is accomplished by using a minimum amount of water in a tightly covered pan.

To use a steamer, fill the pan with water until it almost reaches the bottom of the steamer. Add vegetables and cover tightly when water reaches full boil.

Please note that cooking times may vary greatly due to

the maturity of the vegetables, altitude, and differences in microwaves. Experiment until you find the way vegetables cook best for you.

Foods that are good for you

As a general guide, here is a list of foods that are good for you because they are low in salt, fat, and cholesterol.

lean veal
whole-wheat noodles
skim milk
lean beef
yogurt (low fat)
olive oil
skim milk cheeses
onions
peppers
vinegar
dried beans
dried rice
dried peas
dried barley
chicken (with skin removed)
fish (not canned in oil)
baked potatoes (with little or no butter or margarine)
homemade whole-grain yeast bread (made without salt or baking powder)
natural cereals (without salt added)
beverages that don't contain fat or caffeine

fresh fruits and vegetables
cottage cheese (low-fat or dry-curd varieties)

The facts on fat: good and bad

Forget saturated and unsaturated fats.

From now on, think of fats this way: there's good fat and there's bad fat.

But, you argue, my doctor has been stressing the importance of eating unsaturated fats and steering clear of saturated fats.

Well, now there's a new twist to the story, says *The New England Journal of Medicine* (323,7:439).

Usually, unsaturated fats are better for you than saturated fats. But now you need to watch which kinds of unsaturated fats you eat.

The kinds of unsaturated fats that you now need to avoid are known as "trans" fatty acids — the "bad" fats. These trans fatty acids are formed by a process called "hydrogenation."

During the hydrogenation process, regular unsaturated fatty acids ("good" fats) are changed into a different form. Instead of being in liquid form at room temperature, they are changed into solid form. (This is kind of like ice and water — the same substance in two different forms.)

The new, solid form of these unsaturated fatty acids is referred to as "trans" or "hydrogenated," and they are used in baking products such as margarines and shortenings.

So, you say, ... what's the problem?

Well, here's the clincher.

The effect that these "bad" unsaturated fatty acids have on your cholesterol level is worse than the effect of saturated fatty acids.

Trans fatty acids ("bad" fats) raise levels of LDL serum cholesterol ("bad" cholesterol) and lower the levels of HDL serum cholesterol ("good" cholesterol).

This produces the highest — and the unhealthiest — ratio of total cholesterol to HDL cholesterol. And that high ratio is a huge risk factor for coronary heart disease.

In the typical American diet, 2 to 4 percent of the calories come from these dangerous "bad" fatty acids.

Researchers suggest that it would be a good idea for people who have an increased risk of atherosclerosis (hardening of the arteries) to avoid a high intake of "bad" fatty acids.

One way to avoid a high intake of "bad" fatty acids is to read labels very carefully.

Look for the difference in fats that have been "partially hydrogenated" and those that have been "completely hydrogenated."

The partially hydrogenated fats are the "trans" fatty acids—avoid them. However, the completely hydrogenated fats are not "trans" fatty acids. Eat these in moderation.

Regular unsaturated fatty acids ("good" fats) that haven't been hydrogenated at all are your best bet.

Try to use liquid vegetable oils instead of hardened vegetable oils.

And, as always, try to keep your total fat intake below 30 percent of your daily intake of calories.

How to eat less fat

Saturated fats, found in red meats and dairy products, should be reduced to less than 10 percent of total calories. Unsaturated fats, such as fish and vegetable oils, may constitute as much as 10 percent of total calories. Your entire fat intake should be less than one-third of your total daily calories.

- Eliminate or drastically reduce consumption of egg yolks, organ meats and most cheeses.
- Reduce your consumption of butter, bacon, beef, whole milk, cream, chocolate, almost any food of animal origin, hydrogenated vegetable shortenings, coconut oil and palm oil.
- Use monounsaturated oils like olive oil or peanut oil, or polyunsaturated oil like corn, safflower, sesame seed, cottonseed, soybean or sunflower oils. Use soft margarine instead of butter.
- Never eat any combination of beef, lamb and pork more than three times per week. Choose lean cuts of meat and cut off all visible fat before cooking.
- When preparing chicken or turkey, be sure to cut off the skin before cooking because much of the fat is contained in the skin. Eat the light meat because it contains less fat than the dark meat.
- Eat smaller portions of meat by using dishes that combine meat with vegetables, (especially legumes like beans) pasta or grains.
- Avoid duck, goose, gravies, sauces, casseroles, pot pies, croissants, fried fast foods, prepackaged cake mixes, bis-

cuit mixes, or pancake mixes, ice cream, whole milk, evaporated milk, sweetened, condensed milk, artificial or non-dairy creamers, and bacon bits.

Before changing your eating habits

Evaluate your present eating habits. Note how many high-sodium, high-calorie and high-cholesterol foods you eat on a daily basis. Look for ways to improve your diet and make a commitment to yourself that you will try to improve your health through your diet.

Consider the effects dietary changes may have on your body. Also, consider the effects a drastic change in eating habits may have on your mind and emotions.

First, don't overdose on fiber. Your body has had years to adjust to the lack of fiber in the typical American diet, and it may take a few days or weeks to become adjusted to higher levels of fiber.

If you have a problem with too frequent elimination or flatulence, cut back a little on high-fiber foods like bran muffins and bran bread. Substitute foods which contain adequate but lighter fiber, like oatmeal, brown rice or bread made with half whole-wheat flour and half unbleached, white flour. Each person is unique, so you may have to experiment to find out how much fiber is right for you.

Secondly, if a total change in eating habits is too hard, gradually change your habits by substituting whole-grain cereals for bacon or sausage at breakfast, making sandwiches with whole-wheat bread, or pulling the fat-laden skin and breading off of deep-fat fried chicken. Many people can move in little steps toward a much more healthy diet.

Your approach to eating the foods that are best for your health needs to be continued throughout your life. By slowly making changes, you may be able to live with them for a longer time. Sometimes, drastic changes in diet are too difficult, and the person completely reverts back to his old eating habits.

Learning what foods are beneficial and what foods should be avoided is the first step. If you are only able to follow the following dietary recommendations in half of the foods you eat, you will still receive a substantial benefit. The more that the recommendations are followed, the greater will be the benefits. Even one step in the right direction will be helpful in improving your total health.

At home or in a restaurant, try to eat foods that are lightly cooked: broiled, steamed, roasted or baked in their own juices. Raw fruits and vegetables are often the best selection.

Drink enough water each day to produce a quart of light colored urine. Water is necessary for regular bowel movements, to help prevent kidney stones, to protect us from disease and to prevent dehydration. Drinking "hard" certified pure spring water is recommended.

Also, older people need to be especially careful to drink enough water each day, because many elderly people lose their sense of thirst, reports a recent study in *The New England Journal of Medicine*. Since they may not feel thirsty or uncomfortable, older people can become dehydrated.

In the next chapter, we'll zero in on cholesterol and plaque, that fatty, white stuff in arteries, and what you can do about it.

CHAPTER 3

Cholesterol — The Inside Story

Here is one way to describe cholesterol: a waxy substance found in fats that are usually derived from animal sources.

The news media have reported quite a lot about the dangers of cholesterol. But it is difficult to look at a big juicy steak and think that it contains "a waxy substance ..." that could clog your arteries and lead to heart disease.

But what does all this mean?

In this chapter, we'll outline the information you need to know about cholesterol. Also, we'll begin to describe the steps that may help you bring your cholesterol levels to within healthy standards and maintain them that way.

Priming the pump

To understand the dangers of cholesterol, it is necessary to understand a little bit about the circulation system.

About every second, from before you were fully developed in the womb to the instant you die, your heart beats.

With every beat, the heart acts like a super pump, pushing blood through your veins and arteries.

Every cell in the body is totally dependent on the oxygen and nutrients carried by the blood as it surges through the body.

By the time it gets to these individual cells, blood must pass through arteries and veins that are so tiny, only one molecule of blood can pass through at a time.

With this information in mind, it is not difficult to imagine why a waxy substance that can build up on the walls of blood vessels can be very, very damaging to the circulation system.

This information is brought more closely into focus when you realize that the heart depends on blood vessels to "feed" itself.

All the blood in the body eventually must pass through the major blood vessels in the heart.

If any of these passageways becomes blocked, the heart begins to suffer. And a sick heart cannot efficiently circulate blood throughout the body.

The need for cholesterol

There are several different kinds of cholesterol. We will describe these different kinds to you in a moment.

But first, let's look at how your body turns that nice, fatty steak into a heart-threatening substance.

Understand that cholesterol is a necessary ingredient in the mix of substances that the body uses to build and repair itself.

Cholesterol is a building block in virtually every cell in the body. The problem arises when the body gets too much of a necessary item.

The liver on its own produces a certain amount of cholesterol.

The liver also extracts cholesterol indirectly from foods through the bloodstream.

When a person eats a diet high in fiber and vegetables and low in fats, the liver does not have a source of contributed cholesterol, so less of this waxy substance is likely to end up in the bloodstream.

But if a person eats lots of animal fats (like real butter and cream, fatty cuts of pork and beef) and certain vegetable fats (including palm oil and coconut), there is plenty of the bad types of cholesterol for the liver to throw out into the bloodstream.

The storage problem

The blood carries a certain amount of cholesterol that is needed in the cells. The body uses cholesterol to make cell membranes, hormones and bile acids and for several other functions.

As the blood circulates, the cells take what they need. But excess cholesterol, not used by the cells, must go somewhere.

Some of the excess cholesterol is excreted as part of the body's normal waste products.

But some of the excess goes into storage. It's this stored

cholesterol that causes trouble.

Some of the stored cholesterol builds up as a kind of "plaque" on the walls of blood vessels. The damage is done when the plaque builds up to the point where blood flow is slowed or even blocked. Plaque also weakens the artery walls.

At the very end of the cycle, some of the cholesterol ends up back in the liver where it is converted into bile and eliminated from the body.

It makes sense that reducing cholesterol levels will also improve your heart's health.

According to the Coronary Prevention Trial at the Lipid Research Clinic, each 1 percent drop in the serum cholesterol level can lower the risk of having a major heart attack by 2 percent.

That means that a 5 percent drop in blood cholesterol levels should reduce coronary heart disease rates by as much as 10 percent. These are significant figures when dealing with the top killer in the U.S. — heart disease.

Packaging the fat

As we mentioned before, there are several different types of cholesterol, fat and protein combinations in the body.

These combinations are important because neither cholesterol nor fat can be dissolved in a liquid. Most fat will float. This would seem to make it difficult for the blood to transfer cholesterol to the cells.

But when cholesterol works together with protein and

fat, the body can make little cholesterol packages that are easily moved through the bloodstream.

These packages are called lipoproteins. They are made up by wrapping the cholesterol and fat with a waterproof protein "skin."

When people talk about good and bad cholesterols, they are really talking about different types of lipoproteins. Medical researchers classify these lipoproteins — a protein combined with fat and cholesterol — according to their density.

Why would one lipoprotein have a greater "density" than another?

Scientists describe density based on the amount of triglycerides (fats and cholesterol) in the lipoprotein in proportion to the amount of protein.

The four kinds of fat packages

There are four types of lipoproteins: chylomicrons, very-low-density lipoproteins (VLDL), low-density lipoproteins (LDL), and high-density lipoproteins (HDL).

- Chylomicrons: these are the biggest lipoproteins, but they have the lowest density.

  In the body, the most important function of chylomicrons is to transport dietary fat and cholesterol from the intestine to the rest of the body.

  Chylomicrons also are very important because they help the body absorb fat-soluble vitamins such as vitamin A and vitamin E.

- Very-low-density lipoproteins (VLDL): these are made up of 10 to 20 percent cholesterol.

  The amount actually changes according to age and sex. You may view VLDL as a kind of pre-LDL because VLDL is the substance used by the liver to produce LDL, the "bad" kind of cholesterol.

- Low-density lipoproteins (LDL): these are the lipoproteins that many health writers refer to as "bad cholesterol." When blood test results show high cholesterol, it usually means that the patient has a high amount of LDL. This lipoprotein contains about 60 to 70 percent of the cholesterol in the bloodstream.

  These lipoproteins are literally high cholesterol bombs ready to go off and coat your blood vessels with plaque. That's because LDL serves as a very efficient transporter, carrying cholesterol to the cells of all organs.

- High-density lipoproteins (HDL): yes, Virginia, there is a "good" cholesterol. Or, if we are going to use correct terminology, there is a "good" lipoprotein.

  HDL contains somewhere between 20 to 30 percent of the total serum cholesterol. Research shows that people with high levels of HDL are at low risk for developing heart disease.

  While scientists are not entirely certain about the role HDL plays in the bloodstream, they surmise that HDL transports cholesterol out of the blood and back to the liver where the cholesterol is excreted from the body.

  In other words, a person whose HDL level is high, and bad cholesterol levels are low, will literally be cleaning out his blood vessels.

Young and old affected

First of all, do not assume that cholesterol is only an older person's problem. Deposits of built-up cholesterol have been found in patients as young as 19.

If you don't know what your cholesterol level is, you are also at risk because you are dealing with a big unknown.

The Adult Treatment Panel commissioned by the National Institutes of Health's National Cholesterol Education Program has recommended that all individuals over age 20 should know their cholesterol levels.

Because cholesterol cannot be felt, you may not have any idea that your cholesterol levels are too high until you have already developed serious heart trouble.

To prevent this, the American Heart Association recommends that a physician check your blood cholesterol levels and other heart risk factors at least once every five years.

If you are on a program to lower your cholesterol, you may want to have your level checked more often. That way, you can fine-tune your eating and exercise habits to significantly reduce dangerous levels of cholesterol.

The numbers to look for

Once you know your cholesterol levels, what do they mean? Many times you will be given a single number. According to the American Heart Association, this is what that number means:

- Desirable: less than 200
- Borderline high: 200 to 240
- High: more than 240

The numbers are measured in milligrams of cholesterol per deciliter of blood volume.

If the number you are given is less than 200, it is unlikely that cholesterol is a major problem. However, cholesterol levels should be rechecked every five years.

Also check to see if you have other heart risk factors. These include high blood pressure and smoking.

If your cholesterol is considered borderline, you have a heart disease risk factor that is roughly twice as high as an individual whose blood cholesterol level is well below 200. Most likely, your doctor will recommend a cholesterol-reducing program for you.

A high-risk classification — a number over 240 — means that you are at high risk for heart disease. More testing will be necessary to determine what you need to do to bring down this dangerously high result.

Into the mouths of babes

Many would agree that dangerously high cholesterol levels are best prevented by good nutritional attitudes started at a young age. Infants born today will have the benefit of all the current research and discussion, but only if parents teach these facts to their young and give them a diet based on these principles.

Unlike baby fat, high cholesterol is *not* something a child will outgrow. If a young person has high blood cholesterol, he has two strikes against him:

First, cholesterol naturally tends to increase with age, so high cholesterol in a young person makes even higher levels more likely later on.

Second, food habits started early are the most difficult to change. How many of us still "clean our plates" even if they contain more food than we wanted, including items we know are bad for our diets?

Unfortunately, experts estimate that one in four U.S. children are affected by high cholesterol.

What can you do if you have children in your family?

Follow the same principles for them that you do for yourself, being aware that the children's calorie and calcium needs will probably be higher than your own.

Recommendations in this guide concerning substituting low-fat items for fatty ones and eating plenty of fiber, especially oat bran, are good for children, too. You may want to supplement what you have learned here with a good book on children's nutrition.

Be sure to select a guide that has been written recently. Older ones may not contain all the nutritional discoveries that have been made in the last five to 10 years.

Can I blame Mom and Dad?

Many, after they are told they have unacceptably high blood cholesterol levels, begin thinking about their family history. A heart attack suffered by a father and family discussions about "Aunt Sue's heart condition" suddenly take on new meaning.

Could it be that an unacceptably high cholesterol level, and its subsequent effect on the heart, is actually passed down through the family?

One doctor says that as many as one out of 20 patients has inherited this tendency to have high cholesterol.

What is particularly important in this case is the possibility that a person has had too much cholesterol circulating in the bloodstream for most of his life. That means there is a much greater risk that cholesterol has already significantly built up in the body.

When heredity is suspected in a case, a doctor may have to be particularly aggressive in trying to bring the blood cholesterol level down. He may also want to go ahead and test other family members, even those that are very young.

By finding out early that someone is likely to have cholesterol problems, the overall cumulative problems may be reduced.

Are drugs needed?

It goes without saying that if you and your doctor agree that you need to use medication to help bring down dangerously high levels of cholesterol, you should follow your physician's instructions precisely.

Due to the potential damage to your heart, cholesterol is not a health factor that should be taken lightly.

However, if your personal physician recommends drugs

to reduce your cholesterol, find out why he thinks a diet therapy alone won't work. You may want to seek a second opinion.

Dr. John LaRosa, who works with the Johns Hopkins University Lipid Research Clinic, has said: "Physicians may not rely on diet therapy in part because our medical education has not trained most of us well in nutrition and compliance issues."

Even if you do choose to use drugs in this important health battle, remember that diet is still important.

"Drugs are not a substitute for diet," LaRosa said during a panel discussion reported by the U.S. Department of Health and Human Services. "In fact, a high-saturated-fat diet can negate some of the effects of drug treatment.

"When patients combine a proper diet with drug treatment, the beneficial effect is additive," the doctor said. "Patients who need drug therapy may have to take less medication to reach their goal if they adhere well to a diet."

Keep in mind that drug therapy may not be easy because of some of the side effects noticed by some patients on cholesterol-reducing medications.

These side effects include stomach upset and constipation. Your doctor may recommend certain combinations of antacids and other stomach remedies to lessen these effects.

Remember that eating a diet high in fiber may be the best thing you can do to reduce gastrointestinal difficulties.

In the next chapter, we'll consider specific ways for you to take control of your cholesterol levels, including some pleasant ways.

CHAPTER 4

How to Cope with Cholesterol

Change your eating habits to lower cholesterol

You can make a big change for the better in your blood cholesterol levels just by changing your eating habits. Eating a well-balanced diet is the easiest and least expensive method to reduce cholesterol.

Your goals should be to lower saturated fat intake, which accounts for 40 percent of our daily calorie count. But be careful to keep on getting proper nutrients. Lower your dietary cholesterol, found in meats, dairy products and animal fats; and count calories. (Fat people are more likely to have higher cholesterol levels than normal-weight people.)

Below are some guidelines to help you choose the healthiest foods to eat.

Dairy products: Choose skim milk instead of whole milk; low-fat plain yogurt instead of fruit yogurts made with whole milk; low-fat cheeses (farmer's, mozzarella), and ice milk or sherbet instead of ice cream. Limit egg yolks to less than three per week; use egg whites in place of whole eggs in recipes.

Meats and seafood: Think lean. Choose chicken, turkey, and well-trimmed cuts of lean beef. Eat at least two servings of fish per week. Fish from deep, cold waters are best because they're high in essential omega-3 oils. Fresh or frozen fish are better than canned. But if you eat canned fish, choose fish packed in water, not oil.

Fruits and vegetables: Eat three servings of fresh fruits daily (except coconuts). Avoid fruit canned in heavy syrup. Read the labels on jams and jellies and choose a low-sugar product. Most vegetables and preparation methods are fine, but avoid avocados, olives, cheese, cream and butter sauces. Restrict starchy vegetables, such as potatoes.

Cereals, nuts, breads: Most hot and cold packaged cereals are fine, but watch the sugar and salt content. Also check the labels and buy those that are highest in dietary fiber, vitamins and minerals (remember that dietary fiber is not the same thing as crude fiber). Use pecans, walnuts and peanuts sparingly. Avoid hydrogenated peanut butter. Choose whole-grain breads, and avoid commercially baked goods, such as cakes and pastries, which are loaded with fat. Instead of egg noodles, choose pastas and rice.

The above guidelines are from *Postgraduate Medicine* and are based on recommendations from the American Heart Association and the National Cholesterol Education Program Expert Panel.

How you prepare food also will affect your cholesterol levels. You may freely use vinegar, soy sauce (but watch the sodium) and most spices and herbs.

Cooking oils are another matter. Choose polyunsaturated vegetable oils, such as safflower, corn and sesame oils. Avoid lard altogether. Instead of butter, try polyunsaturated margarine instead.

You might also consider cutting back on your intake of meat protein. Why? Because vegetarians uniformly have lower cholesterol levels than meat eaters, and Loma Linda University researchers now know why.

Protein is the key. According to *Stay Healthy* (3,12:46), plant proteins help lower cholesterol, while animal proteins raise cholesterol. These effects occur no matter what type of fat a person consumes.

Natural ways to lower cholesterol

If you have unusually high cholesterol, your doctor may elect to put you on medication. What follows are general guidelines. For many people, these suggestions will help lower cholesterol naturally, without medication.

- Get regular checkups: it may be one of the most important things you can do. This enables both you and your doctor to keep track of your cholesterol, weight and other items related to good health.
- Maintain your proper weight.
- Get regular exercise (absolutely no less than three one-half hour sessions per week).
- Do not smoke.

  Perhaps one of the most important steps you can take is to change your diet.

Doctors say that many people can expect a 10 to 15 percent reduction of the amount of "bad" cholesterol in the blood by making dietary changes. Others may see a dramatic 30 percent improvement in just two to three weeks when a very strict diet has been followed.

What is the key to making dietary changes work?

Patience, one doctor says. While some people may quickly see remarkable changes, permanent drops in blood cholesterol levels, due to the formation of new habits, are not likely until after six months on a new diet.

Many in the U.S. have already caught on to the significance of dietary changes. According to publications by the U.S. Department of Health and Human Services, changes in diet here have already reduced mortality rates due to heart disease. Our overall diet shows a slight decrease in the intake of dietary cholesterol and saturated fat and an increase in the intake of polyunsaturated oils.

Changing your diet

Here are some practical dietary changes to make:
• Do not consume more than 100 milligrams of cholesterol for each 1,000 calories. Daily cholesterol should not exceed 300 milligrams.
• Substitute fresh vegetables and fruits for processed ones.
• When you do eat out, find out how food is prepared. Always avoid menu items that were prepared with lard, and keep at a minimum items that were prepared with shortening (the palm oil in shortening contains bad fats).

- Select lean cuts of meat. Cut away excess fat, particularly in restaurants where prime cuts are more likely to be used.
- You should get plenty of protein if you limit your daily meat intake to five to seven ounces (cooked weight) of poultry, fish or lean meats.
- When eating chicken and turkey, remove the skin.
- Total fat intake should be less than 30 percent of your daily calories. However, unsaturated fats, such as fish oils and vegetable oils, should make up as much as 10 percent of your daily calories.
- Use low-fat cottage cheese or non-fat yogurt in place of sour cream. These may also be used to substitute for creams or mayonnaise in fruit salads.
- Replace butter with a no-cholesterol margarine. Check margarine labels to make certain no palm oils were used.
- In recipes, experiment with reducing by one-half the amount of fats called for. Make up the difference by adding water.
- Switch to skim milk. Always avoid whole milk.
- Real croissants are practically dripping with butter, even if you add none on your own. It is best to eliminate these from your diet altogether.
- Some think that daily garlic may be good for you by reducing the "bad" cholesterol in your body and by raising the levels of "good" cholesterol. Studies on garlic have used the addition of oil extracted from as many as 10 cloves of garlic per day.
- Use a commercial egg substitute or egg whites in recipes that call for whole eggs.
- Experiment with making your pies with only one crust

(you will save calories this way too.) Try making your pie dough with tub margarine rather than shortening—note that crusts made this way will probably not be as flaky.

* Try substituting ground turkey for ground beef, especially in recipes where the ground beef is mixed with other ingredients.
* Always avoid non-dairy creamers. Most are loaded with saturated "tropical" oils. A better choice: non-fat dry milk.
* Check labels when buying crackers and cookies. Avoid the selections that contain lard or animal fat.
* Use polyunsaturated oils or margarine: safflower, soybean, corn and sunflower oils are all excellent choices.
* Substitute no-cholesterol sandwich spreads for mayonnaise.
* When purchasing pasta, try to avoid those brands made with eggs.
* Use skim evaporated milk in recipes that call for heavy cream. This product may also be used to substitute for whipped cream in some recipes: allow skim evaporated milk to sit in the freezer until ice crystals start to form along the edges of the bowl. Whip into stiff peaks and add a small amount of sugar.
* Emphasize foods high in vegetable proteins such as oat bran, dried beans, peas, tofu, pasta, lentils and rice. For an even greater nutritional boost, select whole-grain or unprocessed products.
* Use no-stick sprays and non-stick pans instead of pans coated with grease.
* When eating out, look for entrees that have been steamed, poached, broiled, stir-fried or baked. Avoid items that

have been sautéed or fried.
• Learn to use spices and herbs for flavoring rather than butter or gravy.

Certainly, it is easy to understand why it is important to know what your blood cholesterol level is and what to do to keep it within healthy limits.

While research into vitamins and other areas offer limited encouragement, it should be evident that no magic pill will suddenly make your high blood cholesterol levels go away.

To accomplish this goal, you must listen carefully to your doctor and make some educated choices regarding your health.

The two most important ones to consider include getting enough exercise and making reasonable changes in diet.

If you follow these guidelines, you may be on your way to meeting at least one of these aims. Your diet should stress high fiber and low fat.

Focus on ways to cut your risk

• Eat fish just three times a week and lower your risk of heart and artery problems, according to Dragoslava Vesselinovitch, D.V.M., from the University of Chicago School of Medicine. Even if you have a high-fat diet, eating fish will help reduce your cholesterol levels, Vesselinovitch says. But eating fish more often will not increase the benefits. Three times a week seems to be the optimum amount.

- Are you eating the right kind of fiber? Americans are increasing the amount of fiber in their diets but only certain types of dietary fiber help to lower cholesterol. Water-soluble fibers, like pectin and guar gum, are the only types of fiber that help reduce cholesterol, Dr. Ann L. Gerhardt of the University of California-Davis Medical Center explains.

Wheat bran contains a non-soluble form of fiber so it doesn't help in the cholesterol battle. Pectin is found in many fruits, like pears and apples. Guar gum is contained in oat bran, oatmeal, rolled oats, and many beans. Increase your consumption of kidney beans, pinto beans, garbanzo beans, chick-peas, navy beans, lentils, all fruits and vegetables and oat bran.

Wheat bran and foods containing non-soluble fiber are still important to a well-balanced diet, but you should know that they aren't involved in decreasing cholesterol.

- A common, over-the-counter laxative has been proven to reduce cholesterol. Metamucil reduced total cholesterol levels by 15 percent in just eight weeks, according to a study by James Anderson, M.D., at the University of Kentucky College of Medicine (reported in the *Archives of Internal Medicine*). Participants took 3.4 grams of Metamucil three times a day and significantly lowered their cholesterol.

Metamucil, technically known as psyllium hydrophillic mecilloid, is made from the husks of blond psyllium seeds. Dr. Anderson decided to study psyllium because it is a water-soluble fiber similar to guar gum, oat gum and pectin. "These preliminary results indicate that Metamucil may help the millions of people whose cholesterol levels put them at risk for coronary heart disease," Dr. Anderson says.

Other products that contain psyllium as the active ingredient are Alramucil, Effersyllium, Fiberall, Hydrocil, Modane Versabran, Naturacil, Perdium, Prompt and Syllact. The article below details more benefits of this husky helper.

A well-known natural laxative that cuts cholesterol

It's cheap. It's easy to get. And it lowers cholesterol.

The "it" is psyllium.

Millions of people have used this common, over-the-counter, natural laxative to get relief from occasional constipation. By taking a dietary fiber called psyllium, they likely were helping their hearts at the same time. Psyllium is the main ingredient in laxative products like Metamucil and Fiberall.

Researchers have found that daily doses of just three teaspoons of psyllium can lower cholesterol levels in the blood by 5 percent and can slash levels of "bad" cholesterol by 10 percent or more. The results are in a report in the *Journal of the American Medical Association* (261,23:3419).

For every percentage point you lower your total cholesterol level, your risk of heart attack drops by two percentage points, the report says. In addition, the fiber supplements can raise the proportion of "good" HDL cholesterol while it lowers the "bad" LDL cholesterol. That also fights your risk of heart disease.

The researchers got these results in experiments with people who had mild to moderate cases of hypercholesterolemia, the medical name for too much cholesterol in the blood.

The 75 people had already been put on low-fat diets to treat their condition. Most received some benefit from just that step alone. In addition to the low-fat diet, half of them took the extra psyllium daily for up to 16 weeks during the experiments. The ones who took the fiber laxative were the ones who had the dramatic additional cuts in cholesterol levels. They took each teaspoonful of psyllium with eight ounces of water.

Besides the beneficial effects of lowering cholesterol, the psyllium supplements had no serious side effects. About one out of six people reported minor discomforts from temporary feelings of fullness with some abdominal cramping. One in 12 had bloating and increased amounts of intestinal gas being passed. Only one experienced a significant laxative effect. "All of these events were transient and minor in nature, and none required discontinuation of treatment," the *JAMA* article says.

The psyllium fiber worked even better than oat bran, according to the report. Overall, eight out of 10 people who took the psyllium (in the form of Metamucil) had lower "bad" cholesterol and total cholesterol levels after eight weeks. That compared to almost no changes in the control group, which had been given a fake supplement called a placebo.

Another study showed that psyllium lowers both total cholesterol levels and LDL cholesterol levels, says the *Southern Medical Journal* (83,10:1131).

The people who volunteered for this study took psyllium twice daily. They mixed three packets of instant Metamucil into a 12-ounce glass of water. The volunteers each drank one glass of Metamucil before breakfast and one after dinner. They also drank a 12-ounce glass of water after each glass of Metamucil.

The volunteers also participated in the American Heart Association diet while they tested the psyllium. The AHA diet helps promote good health by lowering weight and cholesterol levels.

These researchers suggest that psyllium is probably most effective in lowering cholesterol when it is combined with the American Heart Association diet. (You can contact the American Heart Association for a copy of this diet.)

The combination of the AHA diet and the psyllium drinks resulted in a 17.3 percent decrease in total cholesterol in men and a 7.7 percent decrease in total cholesterol in women.

The study also showed a 20 percent decrease in LDL cholesterol in men and an 11.6 decrease in LDL cholesterol in women.

Psyllium is the fiber part of seed husks from the common plant, English plantain. The fiber dissolves in water and forms a kind of gel in the digestive system. Doctors still aren't sure *how* the fiber fights cholesterol, only that it does.

But be careful. Some people are allergic to psyllium, and

they can have serious reactions. Sometimes such allergic reactions can be life-threatening.

A 43-year-old woman ate some cereal containing psyllium, according to a report in *The New England Journal of Medicine* (323,15:1072). Shortly afterwards, she developed swelling and itching around the mouth and eyes and began coughing and vomiting. She recovered after a doctor's prompt treatment. The good news is that such allergic reactions are rare.

Less rare is abuse of laxatives. Some people overuse laxatives, even natural ones like psyllium, resulting in long-term digestive problems.

Be sure to ask your doctor to monitor your progress if you start taking psyllium regularly. More doctors now prefer to use natural means — particularly changes in diet — as the first stage of treatment in lowering blood cholesterol levels.

The good news about apples: Two a day fight cholesterol excess

A French study has found that eating two apples a day can lower your cholesterol level by at least 10 percent, and as much as 30 percent, according to the *Medical Tribune* (30,6:14). Apples long have been recognized as healthful food, but their beneficial effect on cholesterol levels has only recently been discovered.

Researcher David Kritchevsky contends that pectin, the fiber naturally found in apples, is the important cholesterol-lowering ingredient. Kritchevsky, a professor at the University of Pennsylvania School of Medicine, has conducted several studies on fiber and feels that pectin's benefits have often been overlooked, the *Medical Tribune* reports.

Because apples are naturally low in calories, high in pectin and have been shown to help lower cholesterol, Dr. Kritchevsky believes they are an excellent snack and an important part of a good diet.

Some news media reported in 1990 about possible cancer risks from Alar, one of the chemicals used in apple production. Alar's chemical name is daminozide. For a time, many people avoided apple juice, baby food and applesauce even though apples used for these products are never treated with Alar. Daminozide is used mainly to improve the shelf appearance of whole (table) apples. That scare has mostly passed, since few apples now are treated with Alar.

For health's sake, keep on eating apples.

High-fiber cereals for breakfast can help control cholesterol levels

"Breakfast is the most important meal of the day."

That adage is no longer just motherly advice — it's a medical fact. But not just any breakfast food will do.

Your cholesterol levels throughout the day seem to be directly affected by what foods you choose for breakfast, researchers suggest in *The Journal of the American College of Nutrition* (8,6:567).

A nutrition bonus — adults who "break the fast" with ready-to-eat cereal "have significantly lower fat and cholesterol intakes than those who [eat] other foods at breakfast" or even those who skip breakfast altogether, says the report.

The five-year study, called the National Health and Nutrition Examination, analyzed the food intakes of 11,864 Americans.

To determine whether breakfast really is the most important meal of the day, researchers divided respondents into one of these three categories: (1) cereal eaters; (2) breakfast eaters (but without ready-to-eat cereal); and (3) breakfast skippers.

The non-cereal eaters had the highest fat intakes, followed by breakfast skippers.

Among men and women aged 50 to 74, the study indicates that serum cholesterol levels were lowest for those people eating breakfasts that include cereal and highest for those who skip breakfast altogether.

Additionally, having cereal for breakfast seems to help keep cholesterol levels under control—an important factor in controlling your heart-disease risk.

The breakfast skippers apparently ate higher cholesterol meals later in the day, the study indicates. In addition, they might not have gotten the cholesterol-lowering benefits of a high-fiber meal.

Eating a high-fiber cereal for breakfast can result in weight loss, too, according to a study reported in *The American Journal of Clinical Nutrition* (50,6:1303-1307).

Men and women who eat high-fiber cereal for breakfast tend to feel less hungry throughout the day compared to those who eat other breakfast foods or cereals with low amounts of fiber.

Therefore, high-fiber-cereal eaters tend to eat less food during breakfast and lunch, the report says.

Researchers asked men and women between the ages of 24 and 59 to eat a 7:30 a.m. breakfast of orange juice and cold cereal with milk. They ate either Post Toasties (lowest in fiber), Shredded Wheat, Bran Chex, All Bran or Fiber One (highest in fiber of the five).

Three and a half hours later, they ate a buffet lunch.

The high-fiber eaters consumed about 100 fewer calories at breakfast and about 50 fewer calories at the lunch buffet than those who had eaten lower-fiber cereals, according to the report.

The smaller amount of food consumed at lunch was relatively small, but "theoretically could result in substantial weight loss if continued long-term," the researchers conclude.

By the way, a high-fiber hot cereal like oatmeal probably would give many of the same benefits.

Rice bran lowers cholesterol

Rice bran can lower levels of total cholesterol, low-density lipoprotein (LDL) and very-low-density lipoprotein, while raising the amount of high-density lipoprotein (HDL), according to a study in *Lipids* (21:715-7). High levels of low-density lipoproteins increase the risk of heart disease. High-density lipoprotein, sometimes called the "good" cholesterol carrier, seems to help protect the body against heart and artery disease.

Other research at the U.S. Department of Agriculture (USDA) in Albany, California, shows that rice bran lowers total cholesterol as well as oat bran, reports *Science News* (134:20, 308). "Preliminary results show a balanced diet, including 10 percent dietary fiber from defatted rice bran, reduces cholesterol in hamsters by more than 25 percent."

In diabetics, whole rice helped lower cholesterol levels when it replaced potatoes in their diets. "When rice was the major carbohydrate source the very-low-density lipoprotein triglycerides decreased," *The American Journal of Clinical Nutrition* (39:598-606) reported.

The best mealtime cholesterol preventative

Garbanzos, kidney beans and cowpeas are not celebrity foods. But they just might be your best mealtime friends nutrition-wise.

Legumes (or beans) are good sources of iron, magnesium, zinc, protein and several B vitamins, according to the *Tufts University Diet and Nutrition Letter*. In these respects, they are similar to meat and poultry.

Unlike meat, however, "they are practically devoid of fat, free of cholesterol," the *Letter* says. In addition, beans are highest of all foods in soluble fiber, which is now believed to lower blood cholesterol levels and thereby reduce the risk for developing heart disease.

In light of their impressive contributions, beans should

be consumed for nutritional reasons alone. Yet beans are also inexpensive and easy to serve in a variety of ways.

"Legumes combine just as well with vegetables and grains as meats do," the *Letter* says. Also they store easily, and "at a fraction of the price of meat, they are among the best high-protein food bargains you can buy."

The vitamin connection

Will vitamins help you reduce your cholesterol levels?

Many researchers think that several dietary supplements may help protect against coronary artery disease and high levels of blood cholesterol—but primarily when taken in very high doses.

The ones most commonly researched include vitamins E and C, niacin and folic acid.

- Niacin: in studies, this vitamin supplement, in prescription doses, monitored by doctors, has reduced high levels of blood cholesterol and helped those who had suffered heart attacks. In one study, patients who received high doses of niacin had an 11 percent lower death rate when compared to people who had not received the supplement. However, very high doses were used. This type treatment should never be attempted without supervision from a physician. Diabetes patients, and those who suffer from gout or ulcers, should not consider taking extra niacin at all.

- Folic acid: studies have shown that doses as high as

50 to 100 times the recommended daily allowance of this substance can neutralize xanthine oxidase, a substance found in butterfat. This is important because xanthine oxidase can destroy plasmalogen, which protects the lining of arteries. Once again, note the extremely high doses used, and realize that this should never be attempted without your doctor's approval.

- Vitamins E and C: these vitamins help patients who benefit from reducing blood's clotting ability. Research shows that these two vitamins may inhibit blood platelet clumping, which eventually results in blood having less chance of clotting. However, extremely high doses of these vitamins may cause higher death rates.

Details on these vitamin helpers are in the following articles.

A potent weapon

A daily doctor-prescribed supplement of niacin can help lower dangerously high cholesterol levels, according to Mayo Clinic Nutrition Letter (2,10:1). "Daily doses of 0.5 to 6 grams of niacin decrease levels of total cholesterol and LDL [low-density lipoprotein, or "bad"] cholesterol," according to the report. That's 31 to 375 times the officially recommended daily allowance (RDA) for regular, good nutritional purposes.

Niacin, a member of the vitamin-B complex, is prescribed in some cases because it stops the production of LDL cholesterol and helps the body absorb carbohydrates. Experts have known of the vitamin's cholesterol-lowering abilities for more than 30 years and often prescribe it in conjunction with other medications.

In smaller amounts, niacin is found naturally in liver, yeast, lean meat and whole grains.

You might be tempted to self-medicate yourself, but don't. The report offers a few reasons:

- When taken in such large doses, niacin acts like a powerful drug and can cause side effects, such as flushing and upset stomach. The higher the dosage, the more severe the side effects.

- Niacin is not a cure-all. You must change your diet and increase your exercise to lower cholesterol successfully.

- Your doctor may think that another treatment would work better for you.

But take a look at the downside.

Even slow-release forms of niacin in large doses could damage your liver, warn two recent reports in the *Journal of the American Medical Association* (264,2:181 and 241).

Doctors have known for a long time that megadoses of niacin, also known as vitamin B3, can cause liver failure.

But until now, some had believed that people needing large doses of niacin might be better off taking the sustained-release tablets, the kind that dissolve slowly in the body and feed out smaller levels of the vitamin over many hours.

According to the report in *JAMA*, four people developed serious liver damage after taking the slow-release niacin instead of the crystalline form.

Two of them changed from the prescribed crystalline kind to the slow-release kind — one 62-year-old man on his own initiative and a 47-year-old man on a pharmacists's recommendation.

In a third case, a doctor prescribed slow-release niacin for a 50-year-old woman.

All three had been receiving doctor-prescribed treatment of high-dose niacin to lower their high cholesterol levels. They had been taking between 1,500 milligrams and 4,000 milligrams of niacin daily under doctors' supervision.

The fourth said he had been taking one 500-milligram slow-release niacin tablet daily for two months as a supplement without checking with a doctor.

The Recommended Dietary Allowance for niacin is 15 milligrams per day for men over 50, and 13 milligrams daily for women over 50.

Normally, doctors prescribe the crystalline form of niacin, known as nicotinic acid (no relation whatsoever to the drug nicotine found in tobacco).

Niacin in high doses—sometimes 100 or more times the RDA — is very effective in lowering excessive levels of cholesterol in the blood.

The problem is that such high-dose niacin can cause unpleasant side effects, most often skin flushing, especially of the face, and widespread itching.

In addition, a person taking such high doses can suffer liver damage, even while under close supervision of a doctor.

The slow-release form cuts down on the flushing and itching. But it apparently is more dangerous to the liver, in lower doses and over shorter periods of time.

Slow-release niacin tablets are available without prescription in many health food stores and pharmacies.

Such cases point out again the wisdom of checking first with your doctor before taking supplements of any kind.

Be especially cautious about taking megadoses of vitamins and minerals that are far beyond recommended daily needs.

Some megadoses can be dangerous, even deadly.

In a *Saturday Evening Post* article, Dr. Kenneth Cooper also warns about the care that must be taken when using niacin to control cholesterol. He says, "It works in some cases, but you've got to follow patients at least at six-week intervals, because a certain number will develop severe liver problems in conjunction with it. I've hospitalized at least six patients as a result of niacin problems."

Chromium shines as cholesterol guard

Chromium does more than just put a bright shine on your car bumper.

One form of this mineral is a vital nutrient that helps your body turn sugars and fats from foods into energy for cells all the way from your brain to your big toe.

New research shows it also might help lower total cholesterol, especially LDL cholesterol, the "bad" type that clogs heart arteries and raises the risk of heart attacks, says a study reported in *The Western Journal of Medicine* (152,1:41).

Researchers at San Diego's Mercy Hospital and Medical Center studied 28 people who ranged in age from 25 to 80.

They tested a supplement called chromium picolinate, a form of chromium that is believed to be easily absorbed by the body. The daily supplements provided 200 micrograms of biologically active chromium.

Among those taking chromium supplements for six weeks, total cholesterol levels dropped 7 percent, and LDL cholesterol (the "bad" form) plunged more than 10 percent.

The chromium supplements also raised by 7 percent the levels of a protein that forms HDL cholesterol (the "good" form).

The researchers suggest that chromium picolinate supplements might help people lower their blood-fat levels.

The Recommended Dietary Allowance for chromium is not precise. Instead, the RDA is a range of 50 micrograms to 200 micrograms daily.

Some studies show that the typical American diet provides less than 50 micrograms of chromium per day.

The researchers point out that many people might not be getting enough "bioavailable" chromium in normal diets or even in other forms of chromium supplements.

Adding to their worry is the finding that infection, pregnancy, stress, high-glucose intake and just plain aging deplete blood levels of chromium.

Natural sources of chromium include brewer's yeast, calves' liver, American cheese, corn, mushrooms and wheat germ.

Unlike some other mineral nutrients, chromium in its

biologically available form appears to be safe even in amounts several times the RDA, and few problems have been reported with chromium overdoses, says the official "bible" of nutrition, *Recommended Dietary Allowances, 10th Edition,* published by the National Research Council (1989: page 242).

As always, check with your doctor before taking any kind of nutritional supplement.

Odorless garlic: Lower blood-fat without losing friends

Although many physicians turn up their noses at the very idea, garlic for medicinal purposes is making a come-back, according to *The Lancet* (335:114, 1990).

In recent studies, garlic helped prevent heart disease by lowering "bad" cholesterol, raising "good" cholesterol and keeping blood flowing freely.

The problem is, you'd have to eat much more garlic than you (or anyone living with you) could stand. The good news is that health food stores now sell deodorized garlic in pill form.

Kyolic, a product from Japan advertised as "odor-modified, color-aged," apparently lowers blood fats without the odoriferous side effects, according to *Prevention* magazine.

A study at Loma Linda University in California measured the effects of the new garlic on blood fat levels of people with moderately high blood cholesterol levels. The participants in the study were given four capsules, one gram each, of the liquid garlic extract each day.

The "lipid levels" of most patients dropped an average of 44 points after six months, *Prevention* reports. The study's main researcher, Benjamen Lau, says that cholesterol, triglycerides, and low- and very-low-density lipoproteins (LDLs) levels all dropped, while beneficial high-density lipoproteins (HDLs) rose. Apparently garlic inhibits the liver's production of harmful blood fats, he adds.

The key to garlic's benefits lies in its most active anti-clotting ingredient, ajoene, according to Eric Block, Ph.D., of the State University of New York at Albany. Block says the ingredient apparently changes "the surface membranes of platelet cells so they're less likely to stick together."

Lau warns that garlic will not prevent heart disease if your diet still includes a lot of saturated fats. Taken with a low-fat diet, however, garlic appears to be helpful in clearing out arteries. And thanks to kyolic, you need no longer fear clearing out a room of people after taking it.

Avoid this American staple

Other than Mom's apple pie, perhaps no American staple is as loved and cherished as the peanut butter and jelly sandwich. This luncheon standby couldn't possibly be harmful, could it?

Unfortunately there is evidence that peanut oil, which accounts for 80 percent of peanut butter's calories, might lead to atherosclerosis, the blocking of arteries with cholesterol plaque, the *Nutrition Action Health Letter* reports. Studies so far have been limited to animals, however.

These studies will come as a surprise to some who consider peanut oil harmless because it is mostly unsaturated and therefore should not raise blood cholesterol levels.

Yet back in the 1970s, Robert Wissler of the University of Chicago observed that diets high in peanut oil clogged the arteries of Rhesus monkeys more than butterfat.

Wissler's experiments have been questioned because he included so much cholesterol in the monkeys' diets. Researchers have claimed the clogged arteries of the monkeys were due primarily to the cholesterol, not the peanut oil.

Wissler counters that high amounts of cholesterol were needed to simulate the amount people ingest over many years, since atherosclerosis generally requires one-third to one-half of a life span to develop in humans. This is the equivalent of five to ten years in primates.

Wissler also points out that the same amount of cholesterol was used with the other fats tested (butter fat and corn oil) as with the peanut oil. Peanut oil did more damage than the other fats.

On the other hand the *Nutrition Action Health Letter* notes that peanut oil clearly lowers the "bad" LDL cholesterol and cites the low incidence of heart disease among the Chinese (peanut oil is a staple in China). But since their diet includes so little cholesterol and fats of all types, damage caused by peanut oil may be undetectable.

The *Nutrition Action Health Letter* recommends caution.

It is better not to use peanut oil as a staple for cooking until more tests are done. But thankfully the evidence does not yet suggest resorting to "tofu and jelly sandwiches."

Decaf drawbacks

If you drink three to six cups of decaffeinated coffee every day, have your cholesterol checked, recommends *Health Confidential* (4,3:1). Too much decaf can send your LDL cholesterol zooming, putting you at greater risk of heart attack.

The cholesterol-stress connection

One last "peace" of advice: don't get stressed out about your cholesterol levels. The higher your stress level, the more you run the risk of raising your cholesterol levels, says this report.

Stress is fairly easy to define. It includes any unpleasant feeling or emotion, particularly when it involves anxiety or hostility. In short, stress is the culmination of pressures from our modern lives.

The sad fact is that stress also may hamper most of our efforts to reduce our cholesterol levels.

Two studies show this connection. In one, the cholesterol levels of medical students were tested both before and after exams. There was an overall significant drop in cholesterol levels following the tests — in other words, after the pressure caused by the important exams was over.

A similar study showed the same results when tax accountants were tested before and after the April 15 income tax filing deadline.

If that weren't bad enough, stress also has been linked to colitis, headaches, ulcers and high blood pressure. If you are interested in improving your health, and lowering your cholesterol, you must take stress into account.

One way to deal with stress in your life is to keep some kind of personal diary. After keeping this record for several weeks, go back and check to see just what is causing stress in your life.

Once you know this, you can begin to take steps to eliminate the total number of "stress factors" in your life. If these cannot be eliminated, your diary may give clues about ways to lessen the stress these factors cause.

Exercise itself can be a stress reducer. Others have found stretching routines and relaxation techniques to be helpful.

CHAPTER 5

The Fiber Story

With the knowledge gained from research in the last 10 years, you now have available to you a lot of health information that will help you make intelligent choices about what to eat.

Out of all the technical terms and information, here's one solid piece of nutritional advice — eat more fiber.

This may be expanded to say — eat foods that will give you a daily dose of both soluble and insoluble fiber.

How fiber fights diseases

Heart attacks, intestinal cancers, hernias and other diseases are at least partly the result of the American love of a high-fat, low-fiber diet.

Strange as it may sound, the fast food restaurant on one corner may well contribute to the number of patients walking into the hospital on the opposite corner.

It makes sense that a diet that reduces fat consumption and increases fiber will contribute to a healthier life.

In fact, as many as six out of the top 10 causes of death in the United States are diet-related, according to the National Research Council Committee on Nutrition in Medical Education.

What's more, many exciting findings during the 1980s and early 1990s suggest numerous health problems may be eliminated or prevented by increasing fiber consumption.

Research suggests that dietary fiber — such as the fiber found in oat bran — may help in the prevention of heart disease, gallstones, breast cancer, hypoglycemia, diabetes, obesity, depression, appendicitis, colon cancer, varicose veins, ovarian cancer, hiatal hernia, diverticulosis, constipation and irritable bowel syndrome.

Do not assume that fiber like oat bran — or the addition of any other health food — will cure any of these diseases. The idea here is to try to prevent an illness from occurring in the first place.

If you suspect that you have any of these problems, or if you plan to dramatically change your diet as a preventive measure, see your doctor. Only a health professional can say with authority what is best for you.

Two kinds of fiber

Many brans give you what's called insoluble fiber. That's the kind that passes through your digestive system pretty much unchanged from the way it went in your mouth.

As its name suggests, soluble fiber is able to dissolve in

water. When soluble fiber gets to the intestines, it actually swells as it rapidly soaks up water.

While most of us generally lump all soluble fibers into one big category, researchers are a little more specific.

The soluble fibers contained in oat bran include pectin, gums and mucilages.

These all have a well-documented ability to lower lipid (fat and cholesterol) counts.

What fiber does

The story of fiber's value starts in the mouth. Fiber requires a lot more chewing than other, more processed foods.

This extra chewing stimulates the flow of saliva, which in turn opens the faucets for the stomach's digestive juices.

Once swallowed, fiber adds bulk, which helps most people feel fuller and decreases the likelihood that a person will overeat.

Once the insoluble fiber has passed into the intestine, it dramatically reduces the amount of time food spends in the digestive tract. This reduces the possible harmful effects of wastes staying in the system longer than necessary.

This speed has its down side. Some minerals, such as calcium and zinc, may actually be bound by fiber. That means these important minerals have a harder time getting into the body.

These drawbacks should be dealt with, but they should not take away from the other important benefits which fiber contributes to the diet.

One of the most exciting benefits is the reduction of cancer rates when high-fiber products like oat bran are eaten.

While most studies have focused on the mostly mechanical work of fiber (such as helping speed digestive wastes through your system), it is possible that the fiber in and of itself may contain a cancer-fighting agent.

At a meeting of the U.S. and Canadian Academy of Pathology, Dr. Abulkalam Shamsuddin reported that the size and quantity of colorectal cancers in rats and mice were reduced due to the use of inositol hexaphosphate found in high-fiber oats, wheat, rice and corn.

This effect has also been seen by researchers at the University of Toronto.

That means that the roughage itself may be naturally enhanced by the presence of a cancer-fighting agent.

Soaking up the bile

Here is how they work.

Soluble, dietary fibers, including the pectin, gum and mucilages listed above, have been shown to attach to and remove bile acids in the digestive tract. Bile acids are produced by the liver to aid in digestion.

The removal of these acids helps slow the development of micelles, which are necessary for the absorption of cholesterol and other lipids.

Fewer micelles mean less cholesterol and even less

digested sugar can get into the bloodstream.

So, soluble fiber contributes to good health in at least two ways.

1) It can lower the total amount of cholesterol circulating in the bloodstream, especially the LDL or "bad" cholesterol.
2) It can also help diabetics regulate their blood-glucose levels. This could lead to a reduction in the amount of doctor-prescribed insulin needed.

Has all this information been validated through research? You bet it has.

Seeking soluble answers

In one study, a group of 20 men with cholesterol levels over 260 were given diets containing 17 grams of soluble fiber per day.

This fiber was added to the men's diets in two ways: from oat products and also from beans. This is equivalent to one serving of hot oat bran cereal and five oat bran muffins per day or several servings of cooked beans and bean soups.

After only three weeks on this high-soluble-fiber diet, the men averaged a 24 percent drop in LDL.

While HDL or "good" cholesterol decreased slightly in this study, other studies have shown that HDL generally improves, or is not affected, when subjects start eating more soluble fiber.

In another study, both men and women were included in the research. These middle-aged people usually followed diets that were fairly low in fat and cholesterol.

During the study, their already good diets were supplemented with two ounces of oat bran or oatmeal. This adds up to only 5.6 grams of soluble fiber for the oat bran or 2.7 grams for the oatmeal.

Even though this was a relatively small amount, these people reduced their blood cholesterol levels an additional 5 to 7 percent beyond the reduction they achieved by following their low-fat, low-cholesterol diets.

Every little bit seems to help.

Pioneering for oat bran

Other studies were conducted by Dr. James Anderson at the University of Kentucky.

In 1984, he reported that his subjects' high-cholesterol levels fell by 21 percent when they were given three and one-half ounces of oat bran per day for 21 days.

The same doctor also conducted a study at MIT that compared oat bran versus wheat bran usage and their effects on cholesterol levels.

Students who ate 1.5 ounces of oat bran a day saw their cholesterol levels drop by 9 percent. Wheat bran had no effect on blood cholesterol levels, Anderson reported.

Keep in mind that a 9 percent drop in cholesterol readings for healthy college students cuts the likelihood of an early heart attack by as much as 30 percent.

Beyond the general description of the work of soluble fiber on bile acids, researchers are not entirely clear about just how soluble fiber produces all its benefits.

This is because there have been so many different studies done, using different methods and different ways to examine the fiber.

However, many researchers agree that the amount of benefit you will get from soluble fiber, including oat bran, is related to the amount you eat.

When a moderate amount of soluble fiber is eaten each day, a 10 to 20 percent reduction in cholesterol may be reasonably expected.

How oat bran fiber can help you

You have a right to make a certain assumption—if a diet contains generous amounts of bran fiber, it must be good for you.

How right you are. One good choice is oat bran. Oat bran provides the soluble fiber to help reduce high cholesterol levels and the heart problems they bring. And oat bran has the insoluble fiber to help prevent many types of digestive problems and cancers.

Oat bran may also be prepared in many tasty ways and may easily be incorporated into your everyday diet.

Oat bran is good for you for a number of reasons.

- First of all, oat bran is readily available in fairly

unprocessed forms. The less processing, the better it is for you. That means it will retain its important proteins, carbohydrates and vitamins B and E.

- Second, oat bran contains properties that help fight major killers in the U.S. These include cancer, heart disease, obesity, high blood pressure and diabetes. Most specifically, it helps to fight high blood cholesterol, a condition that leads to a variety of health problems.

All this and roughage, too

"But wait, there's more ..." may so easily be said here. With oat bran, there is a lot more.

About one-half of the fiber in oat grain is soluble fiber. That leaves about 50 percent more in the form of insoluble fiber or roughage.

As you may have guessed, insoluble fiber is not able to dissolve in water. It is the indigestible part of the foods we eat.

While it doesn't dissolve in the water in our digestive systems, it can hold and bind water to a certain extent.

Unfortunately, for years, this part of food was often labeled "nonessential." But researchers have gradually increased their recognition and respect of this part of our diet.

In 1980, two federal agencies published dietary guidelines that include information about fiber. These reports were recently reconfirmed. They contained this advice:

"The average American diet is relatively low in fiber.

"Eating more foods high in fiber tends to reduce the symptoms of chronic constipation, diverticulosis, and some types of 'irritable bowel.'

"There is also concern that low-fiber diets might increase the risk of developing cancer of the colon ...."

What about commercial oat bran products?

Beware of high-fiber claims in foods that are commercially prepared.

Many nationally-known companies began marketing "high-fiber" products when wheat germ became popular several years ago.

The recent emphasis on oat bran has created quite a stir, and food companies have begun selling all kinds of "high-oat-fiber" products.

Many of these products either contain so little extra fiber or add so much fat that the good of the fiber is almost canceled out.

The sad thing is, sometimes manufacturers use people's good sense against them.

For example, you would probably say that a muffin would make a better snack than a cookie or that an oat bran waffle would make a better breakfast than a doughnut.

But does that waffle really contain enough oat bran to do you any good?

You can't tell by just listening to the advertisers' claims.
What about that muffin that is now offered at your
favorite doughnut store?

One company's oat bran muffin has more fat and more
calories than a creme-filled doughnut.

Nutritionists at Tufts University set out to see what is
good and bad in commercially prepared muffins.

One of the first difficulties they encountered was a
reluctance on the part of some companies to say what is
in the muffins. One manufacturer of muffins sold in
grocery stores refused to give any exact data at all.

Through laboratory testing, Tufts was able to come up
with the following information:

- A simple, raisin bran muffin sold through a national
  doughnut chain had 418 calories, 13 grams of fat
  and 692 milligrams of sodium. (Keep in mind that
  it is usually necessary to consume several muffins
  just to get the needed dietary fiber.)
- A small, nationally-distributed grocery-store oat
  bran muffin had 220 calories, 8 grams of fat and
  380 milligrams of sodium.
- An apple and spice muffin from a doughnut shop
  had 327 calories, 11 grams of fat and 382 milligrams
  of sodium.
- Another doughnut shop offered a corn muffin. Its
  totals? It had 347 calories, 13 grams of fat and 577
  milligrams of sodium.

These figures should cast some doubt in your mind

about the "healthy" muffins now offered commercially.

Your best bet may be to make your own oat and high-fiber products. That way, you know exactly what is going into them.

Also, learn to read labels and ask questions in food outlets. But be aware that lots of fat, cholesterol and calories could be hidden in the generalized information that you may receive.

One negative study

The news media hopped on a single negative study about oat bran in 1990. But the study itself drew fire because it seemed flawed at best and biased to give predetermined results at worst. It was published in *The New England Journal of Medicine* (322,3:147).

The researchers gave 87 grams per day of oat bran to a group of 20 dietitians and health professionals, with an average age of 30 and none over 49. All were in good health with cholesterol levels below the recognized optimum level of 200 milligrams per deciliter. They compared the results with the same group taking extra wheat bran.

When the professional good eaters failed to show any marked decrease in already low cholesterol levels, the researchers trumpeted the possibly distorted story that oat bran failed to lower cholesterol levels. This happened despite the fact that studies showing oat bran's positive effects outnumber negative ones by about 12 to one.

Oat bran fights back

Oat bran, say many researchers, is still in the cholesterol-lowering business.

A newer study suggests that two to three ounces of oat bran added to the diet every day for about six weeks could reduce your cholesterol levels by 7 to 10 percent.

Funded by a grant from the Quaker Oats Company, a group of Chicago scientists tested the effects of oat bran on cholesterol levels in 140 volunteers, all of whom had high cholesterol, reports the April 10, 1991 issue of the *Journal of the American Medical Association* (265,14:1833).

The volunteers were divided into seven groups. All groups started eating a low-fat diet. Group one, the control group, ate one ounce of a wheat cereal each day, in addition to their low-fat diet.

Groups two, three and four added one, two and three ounces of oatmeal to their low-fat diet. And groups five, six and seven added one, two and three ounces of oat bran to their low-fat diets.

The seven groups stayed on these diets for six weeks. At the end of the six weeks, the volunteers tested their total cholesterol levels and their LDL cholesterol levels. (LDL cholesterol is the "bad" form of cholesterol that contributes to clogged arteries.)

Group one, the control group that ate wheat cereal, showed no drop in cholesterol levels. In fact, the group experienced a slight rise in cholesterol.

The group that ate two ounces of oatmeal daily experienced a drop of 2.7 percent in total cholesterol and a

3.5 percent drop in LDL cholesterol.

The group that ate two ounces of oat bran daily experienced a 9.5 percent drop in total cholesterol and a 15.9 percent drop in LDL cholesterol.

The oat bran had a greater reducing effect on the cholesterol levels than the oatmeal due to the oat bran's higher concentration of a kind of fiber known as beta-glucan fiber.

The study demonstrates that this type of water-soluble fiber, beta-glucan fiber found in oat bran and oat cereals, is effective in lowering cholesterol levels.

The cholesterol-lowering effect is probably most effective when the oat fiber is combined with a low-fat diet, as in the study.

The study concludes that it requires three ounces of oatmeal to achieve the same cholesterol-lowering effects as two ounces of oat bran due to the higher content of beta-glucan fiber in the oat bran.

Anything less than two to three ounces daily results in fewer benefits; and anything more doesn't seem to do any more good.

How to get more fiber

Here are some guidelines for increasing your overall fiber intake:

- Make a good supply of bran muffins and keep them on hand for breakfasts and snacks and to serve as dinner "rolls." Let bran form the cornerstone of your high-fiber diet.

- Eat plenty of fresh fruits. The old saying about eating an apple a day contains plenty of truth when it comes to increasing fiber intake.

- Try to reduce the amount of time high-fiber foods are cooked. Cooking breaks down some types of fibers and may slightly reduce the fiber content of the food.

- Avoid mechanical food preparations which ruin fiber in food before it is cooked. This includes peeling, mashing and grating prior to cooking. Instead, leave the peels on often-peeled vegetables; except potato peels, which may sometimes contain harmful poisons. The peels not only provide fiber when eaten, they also add other important vitamins and minerals. Cut fruits and vegetables into chunks rather than grating them.

- When given a choice, always select whole grains over more processed foods. As Americans become more aware of the need for fiber, food companies are responding with better products. More whole-grain breads are available, and even cookies are being sold with less sugar and more fiber.

- When preparing recipes, try substituting whole-grain flour for one-fourth to one-half of the amount called for. Remember, if you are using oat flour, do not substitute it for more than one-third of the regular flour — it may interfere with the way

things bake.
- Peas and beans are excellent sources of fiber. They have an added plus of being easily stored. Not only do they provide fiber, they are high in protein. They easily form the main dish at a no-meat meal.
- Try mixing mashed legumes into ground beef. This not only stretches the meat, it adds fiber and reduces the total amount of fat eaten. This mixture also makes a good base for Mexican-style dishes.
- Add rolled oats or oat bran to drop cookies, muffins or meat loaves.
- Sprinkle oat bran and wheat bran on cereals, vegetables, desserts and even ice cream.

Beyond bran

Researchers have discovered so many exciting facts about bran in the last few years.

A lot of attention has been paid to that old standby: wheat bran. In recent years, rice bran has begun to attract people.

But the two that will be mentioned here in detail are flaxseed and quinoa (pronounced keen-oh-wa).

Flaxseed: the new wonder grain

Late in the summer of 1989, flaxseed began to create a

stir among nutritionists. Early research indicates that this small, dark grain has twice the soluble fiber of oat bran and 10 times the omega-3 fatty acids of fish.

Omega-3, as you will recall, is the fatty acid that has been shown to lower blood cholesterol and reduce the possibility of other heart problems.

Flaxseed may also be helpful in treating arthritis, asthma, migraines and some skin diseases. It may help prevent colon and breast cancer.

But don't throw out your oat bran in favor of flaxseed. The "new" seed on the market has its problems — it spoils quickly, and the longer it sits, the more rancid it tastes.

Several major bakeries are trying to bypass this problem by milling flaxseed into flour, then using it to make bread.

Another problem affects the elderly. While older people seem to do okay metabolizing omega-3 from fish sources, older systems have some trouble efficiently using omega-3 from flaxseed.

Quinoa: grain from the Andes

Another grain has been used for centuries among the descendants of the Incas who live in the Andes Mountains. Quinoa, as this grain is called, has only been available in the U.S. for a few years.

This millet-like grain is unusually high in protein. Some varieties have more than 20 percent. It averages 16.2 percent protein compared to 14 percent for wheat and 7.5 percent for rice.

What's more, it has protein properties similar to milk with an amino acid balance close to the ideal. In other words, this grain is a complete protein and does not need to be combined with another food for the body to make use of it.

It also contains starch, sugars, fiber, minerals and vitamins. In some parts of the country, quinoa is available in supermarkets and health stores. In others, ask your grocer to order it for you. At least one major distributor includes a recipe book with the grain.

Another great bran

Oat bran and wheat bran aren't the only bran you should be eating. New studies have shown that rice bran is more effective than wheat bran in providing bulk and protecting against colon cancer. Like oat bran, rice bran is also effective in lowering total cholesterol.

Rice bran is "nutritious, has a light, slightly sweet taste, is a good source of protein and iron, and yet is low in calories and sodium," says Doug Babcock in *Cereal Foods World* (32:8, 538). In addition, it causes few allergic reactions, and it is easily digestible, he said.

Rice is also cholesterol-free and "contains only a trace of fat," explains Cornell University's *Consumer News*. "Rice is an excellent source of complex carbohydrates and provides thiamine, niacin, riboflavin, iron, calcium, fiber, phosphorus and protein," *Consumer News* continued.

"It has long been known that the bran layers of the rice

kernel contain the highest concentration of nutrients," Babcock notes. "To gain the most food value, brown rice, which contains the bran layers, was the obvious choice. In fact, until recently, that was the only way we could enjoy the benefits of rice bran."

Now stabilized rice bran is available separately and can be added to your daily diet.

Some cautions

A 75-year-old man must have thought, If a little oat bran is good, a lot is better.

After he suffered a week without bowel movements and increasing abdominal pain and frequent vomiting, surgeons at a Connecticut hospital opened up his lower intestine and found a 2-foot-long plug of "vegetable matter" that completely blocked his small bowel, according to a report in *The New England Journal of Medicine* (320,17:1148).

After they removed the mass, the man went home in three weeks.

A week before he had to check into the hospital, the man had begun eating 60 grams (a little over two ounces) a day of oat bran in the form of oat bran muffins.

Six years before that, the man had part of his intestine removed because of diverticulitis.

Some inside scars from that operation, along with the "excessively high dose" of oat bran and the suddenness of the high dose without any gradual increase, probably caused the man's problem, the doctors speculate.

"We suggest that caution be exercised in the prescription of large doses of bran for the patient who has had abdominal surgery," the doctors advise.

A daily maximum intake of between 10 to 25 grams (under a half-ounce up to just under one ounce) would be better for people with past surgeries or other digestive tract problems, the report says. They advise a low-dose, breaking-in period first.

CHAPTER 6

The Health Benefits of Water

What about this health 'food'?

Since the creation of the world, water has been known as a staple of life. It is still one of the best secrets to overall health.

This is especially true as we age. Yet, many elderly people lose their sense of thirst, reports *The New England Journal of Medicine*. According to the study, older people must be particularly careful to drink eight glasses of water each day even though they may not feel thirsty or uncomfortable.

Water helps your body in many ways. It is necessary for regular bowel movements, it helps prevent kidney stones, it protects the body against disease, and it helps to regulate body temperature. In addition, drinking lots of water will avoid high concentrations of prescription drugs in the kidneys and prevent dehydration.

It is remarkable that so many benefits can come from so inexpensive and plentiful a source. Here's to your health!

If older folks generally don't drink enough water, they especially don't drink enough water with their medicines, says a pharmacist specializing in problems of over-age-50 patients. Maybe doctors should write prescriptions for water to make sure their older patients get enough liquid, suggests Madeline Feinberg in *Senior Patient* (1,4:26).

"All medications, including liquids, need to be taken with a half to a full glass of water," she says. "This will help the medication dissolve more quickly in the stomach and be more readily absorbed. It will also reduce any stomach irritation from the drug."

Some elderly patients even try to drink less water, thinking they are "helping" their medicines. "Some people think that if pills are supposed to get rid of excess fluid, then decreasing fluid intake will be that much better!" the pharmacist writes.

Sometimes, older patients try to overcome loss of bladder control (incontinence) by drinking less water. Drinking less water is nearly always harmful, the article indicates, except for the few seniors who are on doctors' orders to reduce their fluid intake.

Water also holds down urinary tract infections by keeping the bladder well-flushed. In addition, it makes the best and cheapest diet drink available. Drinking water makes you feel full with zero calories.

Water smooths out skin and prevents tiny wrinkles from forming. "In fact, water is probably the best 'anti-aging vitamin' we have for skin," the article says.

But water means water, not other beverages like coffee, tea, soft drinks or even fruit juices, the pharmacist says. "These (other) beverages may contain caffeine, may be high in sugar and calories, or may interfere with drug action," the article concludes.

Cheapest 'health food'

Water may well be the cheapest and most readily available health "food." But, because it is so simple and obvious, many people might overlook its many benefits.

When you consider the fact that more than 60 to 70 percent of an adult's body is made up of water, it's difficult to miss the importance of this substance.

And the body is continuously losing water. Sweat is the most obvious avenue by which water takes its leave. But, the very act of breathing also throws water off. In fact, you lose about a pint of water every day as you exhale.

At times when the body does not get enough water, it cannot rid itself of wastes as easily as when it is fully hydrated. Certain wastes in the body, including urea, lactic acid and uric acid, must be dissolved in water before they can be eliminated.

That means that when you don't drink enough water, your body cannot easily remove these wastes. Thus, toxins build up, possibly damaging the kidneys.

Water is also important for these reasons:

- It helps prevent water retention: The body hangs onto water when it realizes that enough is not being taken in.
- Weight loss: Water is necessary before the body can metabolize fat. Also, water retention will inflate your weight.
- Joint health: Water is part of the system the body uses to lubricate the moving parts of joints.
- Temperature: Water helps the body regulate temperature. The most important way is through sweat: when sweat forms on the skin, condensation helps cool the body.
- General health: Water helps to maintain various chemical balances in the body needed for good health.

Water, water, everywhere — Really?

Where should you get your water? This is a very important question.

When water is treated in modern facilities, methods that keep water free from harmful germs may also leave chlorine and chlorinated hydrocarbons in the water.

Chlorinated water increases the rate of certain cancers.

The chlorine itself may contribute to coronary heart disease. While direct evidence for this theory is unavailable, several studies indicate its possibility.

Studies show that the Eskimos, whose diet is heavy in animal fats, drink water made from pure melted snow. This people group is practically immune to heart disease.

In other places in the world, communities with a low incidence of heart disease also have unchlorinated water systems.

Keep in mind that water may also be contaminated somewhere between the treatment facility and your home.

These contaminants, plus the chemical residue from treatment, may be removed by using an activated charcoal filter that attaches to the faucet. Or drink high-quality, certified-pure spring water.

While bottled water may be a possibility, it is a choice that should be made only when your household drinking water doesn't taste good and when the bottled water is itself pure.

These cautions are given for two reasons. First, many bottled waters do not stand up to tests for purity. They are essentially the same as the tap water that is available in some parts of the country.

Second, you come into contact with water in forms other than just for drinking. Your body can absorb contaminates from water in two ways: through drinking and through bathing. In other words, if the water is too dirty to drink, it is too dirty for showering.

Once again, a good filter system may be your best bet.

How much water should you drink? One doctor recommends a minimum of ten 8-ounce glasses of water every day.

Others recommend as many as 14 glasses of water per day for a person who is very active.

However, too much water can be harmful, even causing

"water intoxication." The best advice on how much water to drink, according to doctors who studied the subject, is "enough to produce one quart of urine per day."

Not all fluids are equal in benefits when they enter your body. That is why you should consider avoiding sugary drinks and drinks that are high in caffeine.

These substances may actually cause your body more harm than the benefit it would get from the extra fluid. In the long run, drinking plain and clean water might be your best bet.

CHAPTER 7

Alcohol Problems

Orange juice may not be your drink of choice at cocktail parties. But if researchers at the University of Michigan had their way, a tall pitcher of "OJ" would be mandatory at every party.

The Michigan researchers studied college students to determine the effect of vitamin C on blood alcohol levels, *Prevention* magazine reports. When the students were put on a "laboratory-controlled drinking spree," alcohol was cleared from their blood faster after having taken "5,000 milligrams of time-release vitamin C for two weeks."

Vincent G. Zannoni, Ph.D., and Robert Susick Jr., Ph.D., who conducted the study, say the faster alcohol clears from your bloodstream, the faster you sober up and the less chance you have of contracting liver disease.

They found vitamin C actually blunted the effects of drunkenness. Although counting backwards by sevens was no easier for those who had taken vitamin C supplements, the students could bring their fingertips together better and distinguish between subtle colors.

Based on the study, Dr. Zannoni thinks "vitamin C can

help protect the average drinker from some of the consequences of alcohol consumption." Still, the best safeguard is to drink in moderation. As Zannoni says: "Everyone should probably drink a little less, and get a little more vitamin C."

Sobering up with 'C'

People with an alcohol problem might help their short-term recovery by taking two grams a day of vitamin C, suggests a study reported in *The Journal of the American College of Nutrition* (9,3:185).

Studies about alcohol detoxification — "drying out" — show that taking large doses of vitamin C really helps in clearing alcohol out of a person's system quickly.

In an experiment with 111 New York City alcoholics, three out of four of those who completed a year-long program centered around taking extra vitamins and minerals stayed sober. Regular non-nutritional therapy produces much lower success rates, reports *Men's Health* newsletter (6,8:12).

A Special Amino Acid and Vitamin Enteral (SAAVE) supplement seemed to help keep twice as many alcohol abusers in a sobriety program in California, says the manufacturer, Matrix Technologies, Inc. The findings were reported in the *Journal of Psychoactive Drugs* (1990; 22:173), says the article.

The studies are adding up: special medically-supervised diets that emphasize balanced nutrition dramatically improve chances for long-term recovery from heavy drinking.

The Recommended Dietary Allowance for vitamin C is 60 milligrams a day for people over 50. Check with your doctor before taking supplements.

Alcohol robs your body of a vital nutrient

If you must drink, you'd better stop at two beers, a major new heart study suggests. More than that amount of alcohol daily may spike your blood pressure and may drain a vital nutrient, calcium, from your body, says a report by the American Heart Association. That harmful effect shows up even if you take extra calcium supplements, the study indicates.

"Our study suggests that for the average person, at more than two drinks a day, some bad things start happening physiologically," says Dr. Michael H. Criqui, co-author of the study published in *Circulation*. "Your blood pressure goes up, and you begin to lose the benefits of the calcium in your diet," Dr. Criqui says.

The study shows that non-drinkers and light drinkers who had higher calcium intakes also had correspondingly lower blood pressures, the AHA report says.

But, the study warns, those who averaged more than two alcoholic drinks a day suffered at least two bad effects —

(1) The alcohol seemed to raise their blood pressure, and

2) The drinking also seemed to prevent the blood-pressure-lowering effects of calcium.

Previous studies show that drinking alcohol apparently leads to poor absorption of calcium in the intestines, the report says. In addition, a heavier drinker passes a lot of calcium through the kidneys in urine, draining the body's stores.

Heavy drinkers sometimes have bones that appear to be "washed out" in X-ray photographs, because they lack calcium, the researcher says. That's added bad news for people at risk from osteoporosis, a bone-loss disease that strikes many women and some men over the age of 50.

You can't get around the bad effects of alcohol simply by taking more calcium every day, Dr. Criqui says. "We found that regardless of the level of calcium or potassium in the diet, alcohol still had an independent [bad] effect," says the researcher. "Alcohol seemed to be a much more powerful influence on blood pressure than either calcium or potassium."

The researcher recommends that you eliminate alcohol from your diet. Short of that, he says, you should average two or fewer alcoholic drinks a day. And because a diet rich in potassium and calcium may help reduce blood pressure, he suggests eating several servings every day of fruits and vegetables (containing potassium) and non-fat or low-fat dairy products (containing calcium).

Criqui and co-workers studied 7,011 men of Japanese descent who participated in the Honolulu Heart Study.

Alcohol and the immune system

Heavy drinkers may be ruining more than just their liver. Excessive alcohol intake may severely damage the body's whole immune system, making it more susceptible to serious, even life-threatening infections like pneumonia, according to an editorial in the *British Medical Journal* (298,6673:543).

Heavy drinking over a period of several years may drastically decrease the number of natural "killer cells," the body's powerful defense against invading bacteria and viruses, said the report.

Heavy drinkers have much higher rates of lung infections, including tuberculosis, than other people. The drinking habit also greatly weakens the liver so that "alcoholic subjects may be at increased risk of both hepatitis and HIV (AIDS) infection," the journal said.

Undernutrition — caused by lowered intake of proteins, vitamins and sources of energy — also contributes to lowered levels of resistance to infections among heavy drinkers.

Protecting your liver

Years of heavy alcohol consumption often result in severe liver damage, known as cirrhosis of the liver. Until now, cirrhosis has been untreatable.

But 12 hard-drinking baboons in New York might point the way to preventing and even reversing the deadly disease, according to *Science News* (138,22:340).

Many of the baboons in the New York study probably felt no pain. After all, doctors were feeding the ape-like animals the alcohol equivalent of eight cans of beer a day.

Along with the alcohol, some animals received a diet supplemented daily with three tablespoons of soybean lecithin. Others ate just regular baboon foods, without the lecithin.

Most of those fed alcohol without lecithin developed severe scarring of the liver, including two cases of cirrhosis.

But the eight-beers-a-day group that got the daily lecithin developed almost no scarring, even after eight years of hard drinking, the *SN* report says.

To clinch the case for lecithin, researchers kept on feeding alcohol to three of the baboons but withheld all lecithin. Within two years, all three animals had developed cirrhosis.

Another researcher reported that lecithin apparently heals liver tissue scarred by alcohol. That might mean a reversal of early cirrhosis damage, the report says.

Animal tests don't always translate into human benefits. Researchers caution that people who drink too much alcohol should cut back or stop drinking, rather than seeking some "magic pill" to allow them to continue their substance abuse. In addition, alcohol harms other parts of the body besides the liver.

Lecithin is a natural part of many foods. It is a major dietary source of the nutrient choline. Natural sources of lecithin include soybeans, lentils, beans, peas, rice, cauliflower, eggs, cabbage and calves' liver. It's also used as an emulsifying agent in prepared foods like mayonnaise and chocolates.

Lecithin has been used as an experimental treatment for Alzheimer's disease without much success. Among its unproven benefits are improved memory and lowered cholesterol levels.

There is no official Recommended Dietary Allowance (RDA) for lecithin, although many health food stores sell it in tablet, powder and liquid forms. Taking too much lecithin can result in a fishy body odor.

If you suffer from cirrhosis or other liver problems, check with your doctor before taking lecithin or supplements of any kind.

CHAPTER 8

Allergies

Allergic to your chewing gum?

Food and food additives are known to trigger allergies, but it is often difficult to track down the additives in everything we eat.

A sudden inflammation of the blood vessels can be caused by the additive BHT (butylated hydroxytoluene), found in some chewing gum. BHT is a preservative added to many products like salted peanuts, cake mixes, potato chips and chewing gum. If you develop a sudden skin rash or allergic reaction, be sure to consider all the products you have been eating or using.

CHAPTER 9

Alzheimer's Disease

Alzheimer's is a disease — always fatal — in which the portions of the brain responsible for thinking, memory and routine physical functions are destroyed over a period of a few months to more than five years.

Alzheimer's suspects

Scientists still don't know what causes Alzheimer's disease or how to cure it. But mounting evidence points to at least three environmental suspects that may be involved in the disease process:

- Smoking — Studies show that cigarette smokers get Alzheimer's disease four times as often as non-smokers.
- Aluminum — Some researchers believe aluminum absorbed in the body gets past the brain's protective layer and poisons nerve fibers responsible for memory, thinking and physical activities. Recent studies suggest that cooking — especially with fluoridated water — in aluminum pots and pans results in increased aluminum ab-

sorption by the body.
- Zinc shortage — Low levels of zinc in the body may contribute to senility, since zinc is needed to repair brain cells.

Aluminum suspicions

Suspicions are growing about the link between Alzheimer's and aluminum in our diet.

Aluminum is a "trace element" (*Taber's Cyclopedic Medical Dictionary*, 16th edition, 1989, p.1885) found in minute quantities in food, water and living tissues. But, the body does not require aluminum for any metabolic processes. In fact, aluminum is increasingly under suspicion as a potent brain poison.

Autopsies have revealed abnormally high amounts of aluminum in characteristic "tangles" of diseased tissue in brains of persons who died with Alzheimer's disease.

More suspicions were raised in the mid-1970s when young patients undergoing dialysis treatment for kidney disease developed symptoms of senility. Doctors found that aluminum in the water used in the treatment caused the rapidly developing senility. When they lowered the aluminum below 0.03 milligrams (30 micrograms) per liter, the senility symptoms were quickly reversed, and the patients returned to normal mental states.

Residents of the island of Guam, where the water is high in aluminum and low in calcium and magnesium, have more cases of amyotrophic lateral sclerosis, also known as

Lou Gehrig's disease. That disease also causes senility and leads to death. It is very similar to Alzheimer's disease, especially in the abnormally high amounts of aluminum found in the brain tissue at autopsy.

Some doctors are warning that aluminum in large amounts can be leached from metal utensils during cooking. Experiments in Sri Lanka (*Science News*, 131:73) suggested that cooking in aluminum cookware with water containing fluorides increases the aluminum concentration by up to 1,000 times more than cooking with water without fluorides. Most Americans routinely drink fluoridated water and use it in cooking, and many use aluminum cookware. New evidence suggests the combination may be unwise.

Alzheimer's disease from your home tap water?

That's also why drinking water may be harmful to your health. Aluminum levels in tap water may be linked to deadly Alzheimer's, one of the leading causes of senility in people from ages 40 to 60, according to researchers in England.

As aluminum concentrations in ordinary drinking water increased, the rates of Alzheimer's disease among persons using that water also increased, said the report in *The Lancet* (1,8629:59). In some cases, the rates increased by as much as 50 percent.

The greatest risk, they found, occurred in areas where the aluminum concentrations were greater than 0.11 milligrams (the same as 110 micrograms, or four millionths of one ounce) per liter of water. (One liter is equal to about one and one-half quarts.) Below 0.01 milligrams (10 micrograms) aluminum per liter, the researchers found, there seemed to be no added risks of getting Alzheimer's disease.

Aluminum sulfate, or alum, is commonly used by water systems during the treatment process, the report said. The chemical is added at the water plant as a coagulant to make suspended solids settle out of the liquid.

The amount of aluminum added varies from plant to plant, within certain limits, depending on the amount of solid materials present in the raw water being treated. In many cases, increased amounts of aluminum added to the raw water means that technicians have to use less chlorine to purify the water later in the treatment process.

While much of the added aluminum is removed before the water is pumped to homes and schools, some aluminum remains dissolved in the treated water and is consumed by water users, the report said. Higher levels of aluminum in untreated water also occur naturally in some geographic locations because of mineral deposits in the ground.

The researchers were concerned that the water treat ment process may add to the already high levels of aluminum consumption in most Western countries. In Britain, for example, they estimated that an adult consumes an average of five to 10 milligrams of aluminum each day, occurring naturally in food. But, researchers say, only a small portion of that is actually absorbed by the body internally.

Aluminum-based preservatives in food may add another 50 milligrams (50,000 micrograms) daily. An adult American may get that much or more of the chemical, especially since many people regularly take aluminum-based antacids for heartburn and upset stomach.

While much of that aluminum passes through the body without being absorbed, the British researchers were concerned that water aluminum is much more "bioavailable." That means it is more easily absorbed during its passage through the digestive system. They recommended that water plants use as little aluminum as possible during the treatment process to cut down on the long-term accumulation of the chemical in humans.

The British researchers indicated that they are convinced of a strong relationship between long-term aluminum consumption and increased risks of getting Alzheimer's disease. "This survey, conducted in 88 county districts within England and Wales, shows that rates of Alzheimer's disease in people under the age of 70 years are related to the average aluminum concentrations present in drinking water supplies over the previous decade," the report said. "A positive relation between rates of Alzheimer's disease and water aluminum concentrations was present whichever way the data were analyzed."

Readers may want to call their local water system to find out the concentration of aluminum in drinking water. If it is above 0.01 milligrams (10 micrograms) per liter, some home filtering system may be warranted. In addition, water systems might be encouraged to use less aluminum in the treatment process, pending further scientific study of the potential threat of long-term aluminum ingestion.

Aluminum everywhere?

Aluminum is such a common material in our everyday lives that it is hard to escape ingesting some routinely. For example, various forms of aluminum salts are used in processed cheeses, pickles, cake mixes, salad dressings and baking powder (not baking soda). A form of aluminum is even added to some table salt to make it pour better during wet weather.

Check the labels of your packaged and canned foods carefully to see if aluminum is used in them.

Water itself can be a cure

Some of the symptoms of chronic dehydration can be similar to those of dementia.

That's the dreaded senility and destruction of the mind that comes with Alzheimer's disease and some kinds of strokes.

It's a serious situation, but, in some cases, it can be cured just by drinking water, according to reports in *Gerontological Nursing* (16,5:4) and *Senior Health Digest* (90,12:3).

Simple dehydration — loss of too much of the body's water supply — can bring on mental confusion, disorientation, seizures and other problems.

As many as four out of 10 elderly people admitted to hospitals for dehydration die from complications brought on by fluid loss.

The treatment is fairly simple: drink lots of fluids,

especially water, at least two-and-a-half pints daily, says the report.

Some seniors stay in a constant state of dehydration, simply because their mouths don't tell them that they need water. They don't feel thirsty even though their bodies may be suffering from lack of fluids.

The thirst response gets rusty with increased age, lagging by two or three days.

In other words, your body might need water on Monday, but you might not get the thirst message until Wednesday.

That's bad any time of year, but hot weather raises the danger level.

During hot weather, you need to drink more fluids to keep your body properly cooled and to make up for fluid lost in sweating.

In addition, blood flow to the skin can be 50 percent lower in people over 65, says the *Digest*. That further lowers the body's cooling ability.

To be on the safe side, suggests *New Health Tips Encyclopedia* (FC&A, 1989; pg.13), drink enough fluids to keep the urine a pale yellow in color, not dark. Dark or cloudy urine might indicate you're not getting enough water.

During hot weather, weigh yourself daily, and drink a pint of water for every pound that you lose, whether you feel thirsty or not, researchers suggest.

Check with your doctor about your fluid needs and how best to meet them.

Alzheimer's: doctors wrong half the time

At least half the people who were told they had incurable Alzheimer's disease, a senile deterioration of the mind, were wrongly diagnosed, according to a recent study by Dr. John F. Aita of Midwest Clinic in Omaha. A majority of those diagnosed as having Alzheimer's were suffering instead from a variety of other problems. Some of them could be cured by taking vitamin supplements, the study indicated.

A British study recently reported similar findings about wrong diagnoses that confused Alzheimer's with symptoms of senile dementia (loss of mental capacity, especially loss of memory) caused by other diseases. That same report also suggests some very good news: eating less cholesterol during our early and middle years may cut in half our chances of getting senile dementia during our later years.

In a study of supposed Alzheimer's patients, Dr. Aita found that only 85 of 200 patients had Alzheimer's disease, one of several causes of senile dementia. The other 115 people suffered from a variety of illnesses, including brain tumors and reversible vitamin deficiencies. Most of these other problems can be treated, and some can be cured, Dr. Aita said. There is no known cure for Alzheimer's disease.

The London University study (reported in *British Medical Journal*, 297:894) said that autopsies on diagnosed Alzheimer's victims revealed that more than half of them had died of cerebrovascular disease (CVD) instead of Alzheimer's. CVD is caused, among other things, by cholesterol blockage of arteries in the brain. Such blockage leads to blood clots, strokes, hemorrhages, and resulting destruction of brain tissue.

If we eat less fat and cholesterol, generally, we can dramatically lower our chances of suffering from blocked brain arteries and accompanying senile dementia, the findings suggest.

Alzheimer's usually results in death within a few months or years after the first symptoms become evident. Memory loss is one of its chief symptoms, but an accurate diagnosis should be made by a competent physician, experienced in diagnosing Alzheimer's disease. Some memory loss is normal as people age.

Alzheimer's is sometimes diagnosed in a doctor's office based on the visible signs of memory loss, difficulty in walking, confusion, depression, or loss of reflexes. But Dr. Aita warns that complete neurological exams, done over several days in a hospital, are needed to make a proper diagnosis.

Brain tumors, vitamin B12 deficiency, depression, kidney problems, alcohol-related dementia, and some toxic metabolic disorders can mimic the signs of Alzheimer's disease and cause an incorrect diagnosis.

However, many brain tumors can be removed by surgery. Most kidney problems can be treated or cured with prescription drugs. A deficiency of vitamin B12 can be treated with vitamin supplements, according to *American Family Physician* (36,5:196).

Since the absorption of vitamin B12 decreases with age, older people need to increase their intake of B12 to get the 2.0 micrograms necessary each day. (A microgram is one-millionth of a gram.) Intestinal diseases or long-term use of aspirin, acetaminophen, codeine, oral contraceptives, or neomycin can interfere with the body's absorption of vitamin B12 and cause a deficiency. People with severe intestinal absorption problems should receive vitamin B12 shots. Natural sources of B12 include liver, meat, milk, dairy products, fish, and eggs.

CHAPTER 10

Arthritis

Some current research about arthritis treatment

You may be able to reach into your kitchen spice cabinet for relief from the pain and inflammation of rheumatoid arthritis. Arthritis patients reported "significant relief" from pain after taking less than a tablespoonful of ginger every day for three months, reports Dr. Krishna C. Srivastava of the Institute of Odense in Denmark. Long known as a folk remedy for various ailments, ginger now is being studied in medical trials to determine its usefulness as an arthritis medicine.

The arthritis patients took ginger in two ways: either about five grams a day of fresh ginger root, or from a half-gram to 1.5 grams daily of ginger powder. All reported that "they were able to move around better and had less swelling and morning stiffness after taking the spice," says *Medical Tribune* (30,18:16). No side effects were reported.

Another potential medicine comes from China and has been used there for centuries as a folk remedy. Researchers are planning large-scale trials of an extract from a herb known as *Tripterygium wilfordii hook.*

The Chinese extract "achieved a 90 percent reduction in pain and other typical RA symptoms in 30 patients who were treated for 12 weeks," according to the *Tribune* report. Control patients given a placebo (a harmless fake medicine) recorded less than a fourth as much relief. The main side effects were skin rash in half the patients and mild diarrhea in about a fifth.

Still another natural source of arthritis help is showing up in bark extracts from an Indian tree known as *Dysoxylum binectariferum.* The extract, known as rohitukine, has been shown to cut inflammation and decrease some bad effects of the body's own immune system turning against itself, according to Dr. A.N. Dohadwalla in Bombay. Even high dosages produced no bad side effects in animal tests, the doctor says.

In addition, possible arthritis help may come from deposits of decaying vegetation. A plant extract tested recently comes from some rich peat bogs in Poland. Peat is a soft forerunner of coal.

The refined product seems to cut down on the autoimmune response that, in rheumatoid arthritis, points the body's anti-disease weapons at the body tissues themselves.

The importance of early diagnosis

Many people seem to believe that arthritis is a natural

result of growing old and think that arthritis isn't harmful, so they treat themselves rather than going to a doctor. However, since there are several different types of arthritis, and because of the high death rate in rheumatoid arthritis, a doctor should always be consulted.

Early and aggressive treatment of rheumatoid arthritis is very important. British researchers have found that waiting too long to treat rheumatoid arthritis can be fatal. According to a 25-year study by the Royal National Hospital for Rheumatic Diseases in Bath, England, one-third of people with rheumatoid arthritis died because of arthritis-related problems.

"People really do die from arthritis," cautioned Dr. Theodore Pincus of Vanderbilt University in Nashville. Furthermore, medical treatment within the first six months of rheumatoid arthritis also can prevent irreversible damage to the joints and cartilage, as well as lowering the death rate, the researchers concluded.

Oil for the pain

In gouty arthritis, diet may play a major role in prevention of the painful attacks.

If rheumatoid arthritis is suspected, fish oil may reduce the painful symptoms, says Dr. Edward Harris, chairman of medicine at Stanford University. This is especially effective if treatment with the oil is supplemented with daily aspirin, Harris told *Medical World News*. Then, if the disease is confirmed, standard drug treatments can be started, he added.

Doctors recommend getting the essential ingredients in fish oil — the omega-3 fatty acids — by eating cold-water fish rather than by taking fish oil capsules. High levels of these beneficial oils are found naturally in all cold-water fish. Increase your intake of trout, salmon, mackerel, or cod. Packaged fish oil supplements, available at the store, could cause other problems, such as reducing the ability of your blood to clot. For that reason, most doctors believe the supplements should be used with caution.

People with active, painful rheumatoid arthritis discovered they had less pain, fewer swollen joints, decreased morning stiffness and improved strength in their hands after taking daily "fish oil" pills for nearly six months.

The daily supplement of omega-3 fatty acids also appeared to halt and even reverse arthritis's invasion of other joints, says the report in *Arthritis and Rheumatism* (33,6:810).

Researchers at the Albany Medical College in New York tried "high" and "low" doses of omega-3 oils on the volunteers.

They gave a third group pills containing olive oil, the report says.

The amounts given were linked to a person's weight.

For example, the "high" dose was the equivalent of a quarter-ounce of fish oil per day for a man weighing 180 pounds. That's less than two ounces of fish oil per week.

Women in the study also got amounts corresponding to their weights.

The "low" dose was half that of the "high."

About one person out of every four of the volunteers

experienced fishy after-taste or belching, usual side-effects of taking fish oil capsules.

The researchers suggest that such side-effects are minor compared to side-effects of standard drug therapy for arthritis.

Fish oil supplements can cause increased bleeding times, the report notes.

Those taking the olive oil supplements reported that 24 weeks of vegetable oil failed to ease joint tenderness, morning stiffness or pain levels.

Only the high-dose fish-oil group got significant pain relief, the report says.

The "high-dose" and "low-dose" concepts were defined by the researchers just for the purposes of their clinical trial.

However, other studies have used daily doses of omega-3 oils many times higher than that used in this study, but always with close medical supervision.

Always check with your doctor before taking any supplements, natural or otherwise.

CHAPTER 11

Asthma, Bronchitis

Soy distress

If you suffer from asthma attacks, the villain causing your distress may be as near as your pantry.

Epidemics among dockworkers and residents living near the docks in Barcelona and Cartagena, Spain, have led researchers to identify a new asthma trigger: soybean dust, according to reports in *The Lancet* (2,8662:538) and *The New England Journal of Medicine* (320,17:1097).

Soybeans are a member of the legume family, which includes peas and beans. A common U.S. farm crop, soybeans are high in protein and are used in many commercially prepared foods.

Soy products include soy flour and oil, both of which are used in many food products, from margarine to fillers in canned and frozen meat products.

According to the reports, "extracts of the bean can cause an immediate allergic response."

During one epidemic, researchers found that 64 of 84 adults were allergic to soybean products. For some reason, children under age 14 were not affected.

In another epidemic, 65 patients were sent to the hospital with acute asthma. One died, and nine others needed a respirator to help them breathe.

Experts have known for some time that air pollution and thunderstorms, which stir up a lot of dust, cause asthma epidemics. But, the reports say, the weather was not a factor in the 13 epidemics in Barcelona.

On each asthma epidemic day, however, dockworkers were unloading soybeans. No epidemics were reported on other days.

Researchers point out that the increasing popularity of soybean products may lead to asthma epidemics in other parts of the world.

If you are experiencing unexplained breathing difficulties or allergies, ask your doctor to test you for sensitivity to soy products.

Vitamin C, niacin beat bronchitis

If you're wheezing from repeated attacks of bronchitis, you may need more vitamin C and niacin, says a digest in *Modern Medicine* (57,10:17).

At the same time, a salty diet may be troubling your lungs. People who ate a tenth of an ounce of salt a day were 27 percent more likely to come down with bronchitis than those on a low-salt diet, the report says.

CHAPTER 12

Blood Pressure

A plan to prevent high blood pressure naturally

If you are prone to high blood pressure, are you destined to be forced to take powerful drugs to fight the disease? Maybe not. You might have a natural option that would prevent high blood pressure from ever developing, say eight researchers at Northwestern University Medical School in Chicago.

"Results indicate that even a moderate reduction in risk factors for hypertension among hypertension-prone individuals contributes to the primary prevention of the disease," the report says. (Hypertension is the scientific name for high blood pressure.)

What is blood pressure, and when is it high?

Blood pressure is the force exerted on your blood by the

pumping action of the heart. Blood pressure is expressed in millimeters of mercury (chemical symbol Hg) and measures systolic (upper number) and diastolic (lower number) pressures, as in the "normal" pressure reading of 120-over-80.

Systolic is the pumping pressure of the heart, while diastolic is the at-rest pressure of blood in vessels between heartbeats.

Usually, doctors are more concerned with the diastolic or lower number. Under 90 is considered normal, 90 to 104 is mild, 105 to 114 is moderate, and 115 or over is severe.

You might be able to cut your risk of developing high blood pressure by following these same moderate changes in life-style, the scientists indicate in a report in the *Journal of the American Medical Association* (262,13:1801).

The researchers studied 201 men and women who were slightly overweight, ate salty foods, smoked, downed several alcoholic drinks a day, and rarely exercised. All of them had blood pressure in the "high-normal" range. That means a diastolic (lower number) pressure of from 80 to 99 mm Hg. But, otherwise, they all were healthy.

These prime candidates for high blood pressure agreed to work on better nutrition and to shoot for four goals: (1) lose at least 10 pounds, (2) reduce daily salt intake to less than one-tenth of an ounce, (3) cut back to no more than two alcoholic drinks a day, and (4) exercise for 30 minutes three times a week. Smokers were advised to kick the habit. The researchers encouraged the study participants to stick to a "fat-modified, American Heart Association-type diet."

For five years, the participants—ranging in age from 30

to 44—kept food diaries, visited the doctors regularly, were given blood and urine tests, and had their blood pressures checked periodically. Three-quarters of them exercised faithfully, mostly walking, jogging and bicycling. One out of four met the weight-loss goal, but fewer than two in 10 reduced salt intakes. All said they averaged no more than two drinks a day. They cut their daily calorie intake by an average of 800 calories, a drop of 30 percent. They cut back modestly on saturated fat and cholesterol.

During the same period, doctors kept track of another, similar group that took no special dietary, weight-loss or exercise measures — in other words, just everyday folks who continued to eat, drink and do what they pleased.

After five years, the researchers found that the "do-as-you-please" group had double the rate of high blood pressure as the study group. The nutritional approach also helped even those in the study group who did develop high blood pressure by delaying its onset for a year or more in most cases. Those who lost the most weight experienced the most benefits, the researchers report. On the negative side, smokers were nearly four times as likely to develop high blood pressure as non-smokers, the report indicates.

One in five people in the "do-as-you-please" group developed high blood pressure during the five-year trial, compared with one in 11 in the nutrition study group. That proved true even though most in the study group did not reach their original goals. Just the emphasis on nutrition seemed to help a lot.

Such modest changes in life-style could slash the risks of heart disease and stroke in 1 million people with high-normal blood pressure over the next five years, the researchers believe. "Savings in numbers of cases among older persons would enlarge this potential even further," the report says. The researchers recommend that doctors start aiming for "primary prevention [of high blood pressure] by safe nutritional-hygienic means" in addition to prescribing drugs to fight the disease.

Learning to like a low-sodium diet

A low-sodium diet is one of the basic, natural ways to lower high blood pressure, but many people are hesitant because they think that a salt-free diet is bland. However, researchers at the University of Minnesota discovered that your desire for salt and your taste change when you start a low-salt diet.

"The study was initiated because many participants in earlier studies reported that once they were on a low-sodium diet, many foods that had been acceptable were now 'too salty' or even unpleasant," Dr. Richard Grimm recently announced.

Participants on a low-salt diet compared salted crackers at regular intervals. "The highest sodium content crackers were rated more salty and less pleasant," Grimm said. "The level of sodium preferred also decreased ... these changes in taste occurred early and were evident by the sixth-week visit."

"In questionnaires, men on low-sodium diets reported they were more sensitive to the taste of salt, found many high salt foods to be unpleasant, and stated that the diet was easier to follow the longer they stayed on it," Grimm explained.

This confirms other studies that suggest our craving for salt is a learned behavior — an acquired taste. According to *High Blood Pressure Lowered Naturally* (FC&A Publishing), other studies with twins also show that salt craving is created by a high-salt diet.

It will take up to three months to completely lose the craving for salt, according to Mrs. Dash, a manufacturer of no-salt products.

The average American eats five to 10 grams of sodium, or one-third to one-fifth of an ounce of salt per day. This is much more salt than is needed for bodily functions. Most people only need one-tenth that amount. Many scientific studies show that reducing salt intake, ideally to 500 milligrams per day, will lower blood pressure in most people.

Processed foods, anything that comes in a can, a frozen package or a box, is likely to have salt added as a preservative or flavor enhancer.

Tips to provide flavor without salt include:

- Use lemon juice on food instead of salt
- Use one of several salt-free mixtures of herbs and spices now available
- To spice chicken dishes, add fruit such as mandarin oranges or pineapples
- Marinate chicken, fish, beef or poultry in orange juice or lemon juice
- Use homemade mustard or honey to glaze meat

dishes
- Use green pepper, parsley, paprika or red pepper
- In baking, use extracts instead of salt
- Learn about the many natural herbs, spices and fruit peels that are available

Bran and other fibers lower blood pressure

Daily fiber supplements helped lower high blood pressure, according to a recent study. Systolic pressure, the first number in blood pressure readings, dropped an average of 10 points, and the diastolic pressure, the second number, decreased an average of five points in just three months with fiber supplements, Danish researchers revealed in *The Lancet* (2,8559:622-3). However, people in the control group of the study who took a placebo (a harmless, fake drug) experienced no change in their blood pressure levels.

Your fiber intake should be at least 30 grams each day and should include a variety of fiber types, according to the National Cancer Institute. Good sources of fiber include wheat bran, oat bran, fruits, vegetables (with skins), whole-grain breads, and cereals.

Until modern times, our ancestors ate a high-fiber diet, and many present-day digestive, colon, and bowel problems were rare in those days. Our digestive system is designed to handle a diet that contains bran, the outer fiber of cereal grains. Modern food-processing methods remove much of the fiber from our food, which leads to constipation and other health problems, as well as high blood pressure.

Low-fiber diets have also been linked to heart and artery disease, constipation, appendicitis, colon cancer, diverticulosis, cancer of the large bowel, hemorrhoids, and obesity.

Fish oil lowers 'mild' high blood pressure

High doses of fish oil lowered blood pressure in men with mild high blood pressure, according to a new study published in *The New England Journal of Medicine* (320,16:1037).

"We found that dietary supplementation with high doses of fish oil given for one month lowered blood pressure in men with mild essential hypertension, whereas a lower dose of fish oil, the same amount of safflower oil, or a mixture of saturated and unsaturated oils produced no significant change," reports Dr. Howard Knapp of Vanderbilt University.

The researchers compared the effect of the fish oil (15 grams daily, or slightly more than one-half ounce) with common prescription blood-pressure reducers. "The magnitude of the effect that we found was similar to that of propranolol or a thiazide diuretic in the Medical Research Council trial," Knapp says.

Although these results are promising, the researchers warn that "the clinical usefulness and safety of fish oil in the treatment of hypertension will require further study."

Vitamin C may lower
high blood pressure

Doctors one day might tell people with borderline high blood pressure, "Take one vitamin C tablet every day to get your blood pressure back to normal."

That's because researchers have discovered that vitamin C might prevent healthy people from developing high blood pressure and might even help lower slightly elevated blood pressure readings to normal levels, according to a report in *Science News* (137,19:292)

Checking 67 healthy men and women ages 20 to 69, researchers at the Medical College of Georgia in Augusta found that those with high levels of vitamin C in the blood averaged a blood pressure reading of 104/65.

Those with one-fifth those blood levels of vitamin C — but still within acceptable, normally healthy levels — averaged blood pressure readings of 111/73, the report says. The "normal" blood pressure reading usually is considered 120/80.

Researchers suggest that the vitamin somehow pushes blood pressure down, keeping levels at or below "normal."

That provides a cushion against blood pressure rising beyond healthy levels.

Even people with established high blood pressure may benefit from more C, suggest researchers at Tufts University in Boston.

They checked 241 elderly Chinese-Americans and found the same result: the lower the blood levels of vitamin C, the higher the blood pressure.

Another common thread in both studies: even at the lower ranges of vitamin C measured in the volunteers, none of the people suffered from a vitamin C deficiency.

So the question researchers will be asking is this: are current "minimum" recommended levels of vitamin C (60 milligrams daily) large enough to give this apparent protection against high blood pressure?

Or should people with a tendency toward high blood pressure increase their daily vitamin C intake to around one gram per day, as suggested by U.S. Department of Agriculture scientist David L. Trout?

Check with your doctor first before taking extra vitamin C. Some studies show that taking more than one gram of vitamin C a day can cause kidney stones, gout, diarrhea, cramping and interference with some blood tests.

In addition, suddenly stopping big doses of vitamin C can cause "rebound" scurvy, a serious vitamin deficiency.

You can get vitamin C naturally by eating citrus fruits and dark-green vegetables like broccoli.

Potatoes and bananas may help lower high blood pressure

A low-potassium diet may contribute to high blood pressure, according to a report in *American Family Physician* (41,1:318).

In a recent study, 10 healthy men ate a low-potassium diet or a normal-potassium diet for four to eight weeks.

Those on the low-potassium diet had significantly higher blood pressures after eight weeks than the men on normal-potassium diets, researchers said.

You can add potassium to your diet by eating more fruits and vegetables, such as bananas, beans and peas. Potatoes and potato flour are especially high in potassium.

The estimated minimum daily requirement for potassium is somewhere around two grams, or about one-fourteenth of an ounce.

Other experts urge even higher amounts of potassium for its anti-stroke and blood-pressure-reducing benefits — up to 3.5 grams per day, according to the latest official government recommendation reported in *Recommended Dietary Allowances, 10th Edition* (National Academy Press, Washington, D.C., 1989: page 256).

Earlier studies have shown that a low-potassium diet can also lead to stroke, and researchers plan more studies to confirm their results.

The moral of the story — eat more fruits and vegetables to get more potassium.

If you are taking medicines or suffer from an illness or disease, check with your doctor about how much potassium you should take in each day.

Could a low-salt diet send your pressure soaring?

For years doctors have been telling you too much salt can send your blood pressure soaring.

Apparently, one doctor has changed his mind.

Dr. Brent M. Egan, a blood pressure specialist, told the audience at the recent annual American Heart Association meeting in New Orleans that a low-salt diet may actually be harmful for some people.

He and his colleagues studied 27 men who were put on a very low-salt diet for one week. They then ate their regular diet for two weeks and then repeated the low-salt diet once more.

Many men with normal blood pressure were "salt-resistant," says Dr. Egan, meaning that their blood pressure did not automatically fall when their salt intake was reduced.

In fact, blood pressure actually increased by as much as five points in some men who reduced salt intake, he reports.

Studies have shown that insulin, a hormone produced by the pancreas, in some cases contributes to hardening of the arteries by helping the body produce excessive cholesterol.

Insulin also encourages the body to retain salt in the kidneys, the report says.

Many men in the study had higher levels of insulin, and Dr. Egan suggests that the body may "adapt" to a low-salt diet by producing more insulin.

The American Heart Association recommends that Americans eat no more than one and a half teaspoons of salt a day. (The AHA has no plans to change that recommendation.)

If you are on a low-salt diet — or if your doctor has recommended one — Dr. Egan suggests that you carefully monitor your blood pressure at home. (You can buy blood pressure monitors at your local drugstore.)

Take your blood pressure every day for one week to establish your baseline measurement before starting the diet. Once on the diet, monitor your blood pressure regularly.

If your blood pressure doesn't fall after one to two months on the low-salt diet, talk with your doctor because, Dr. Egan says, the diet "apparently is not helping."

Job demands influence blood pressure

If you've ever suspected that your high-pressure job is bad for your health, you might have been correct.

According to a study reported in the *Journal of the American Medical Association* (263,14:1929), men who hold jobs with high demands over which they have little or no control are three times more likely to suffer from high blood pressure than men who don't.

These workers are also more likely to suffer from physical changes to the heart that could lead to heart disease over time.

Researchers report that the risk of job-related hypertension increases with age.

Foods to avoid

Here are some foods and preparations to avoid as you seek to lower your blood pressure naturally:

canned soup
bacon
pickles or olives
cheese
potato chips or pretzels
salted nuts
french fries
most crackers
canned vegetables
sauerkraut
canned meats
liver
smoked meat or fish
shrimp
luncheon meat
lobster
salt cured ham
herring
pork
sardines
sausage
caviar
pepperoni
anchovies
hot dogs
flavored gelatin
instant cocoa mixes
pizza
most processed food
chocolate milk

"fast food"
ice cream
most frozen dinners
milk shakes
beer
baking powder
tomato sauce
baking soda
most sauces
garlic salt
gravy
onion salt
bouillon
celery salt
ketchup
salad dressings
mustard
cake mixes
relish
pancake mixes
horseradish
muffin mixes
chili sauce
pudding mixes
steak sauce
biscuit mixes
Worcestershire sauce
cornbread mixes
soy sauce
many laxatives

peanut butter
meat tenderizer
MSG (monosodium glutamate)
foods containing sodium bicarbonate
foods containing disodium phosphate
salted butter or salted margarine

The rest of the chapter will elaborate on some of the key dietary factors which affect blood pressure.

Salt: Good and bad news

You may be already preparing yourself to hear that one more flavor you love—salt—is bad for your health. Is there nothing you can enjoy eating anymore?

Salt itself isn't bad for your health. You may remember how your grandparents used salt liberally to cure and preserve meats in the smokehouse on their farm—and no one mentioned high blood pressure back then. And you may know that in the Bible Jesus says, "Ye are the salt of the earth," indicating that even thousands of years ago salt was a valuable commodity for preserving food and stimulating taste buds. The word from which we get our word "salary" comes from the Latin word "sal," meaning salt. Roman soldiers were sometimes said to be "worth their salt" because they were often paid in salt rather than actual money.

Why, then, all the fuss about removing salt from our diets? Why is it so bad all of a sudden? Is this a passing medical "fad"?

Unfortunately the answer is "no" — this is not a passing problem. What has happened is that we have simply "overdosed" on a good thing to the point that it has become a bad thing.

Salt, or sodium chloride, is essential to life. It is an important mineral in the body. Without it we would die. Salt maintains fluid levels between the cells and the blood system and acts as an electrolyte to help chemical and electrical reactions in the body.

However, our bodies are equipped to handle only so much salt. Dr. Cleaves M. Bennett, author of *Control Your High Blood Pressure Without Drugs* (p. 36-37), says, "The quantities of salt we actually eat are a great burden on our systems. It's so destructive. As we eat more salt than the kidneys can readily excrete, over a long period of time, many years, salt builds up in the body.... The body's way to get rid of more of that salt... is to push it out through the kidneys by raising the blood pressure."

The average American eats five to 10 grams of sodium, or one-third to one-fifth of an ounce of salt per day. This is much more salt than is needed for bodily functions. Most people only need one-tenth that amount. Recent studies indicate that some people need as little as one-fifth of a gram (200 milligrams) of salt per day. However, there are exceptions. Hard labor, profuse sweating, pregnancy, and breast-feeding may increase the need for salt up to two grams per day.

Most people will question whether they really consume one-third to one-fifth of an ounce of salt per day, but

processed foods that North Americans eat are usually filled
with salt. Any food that comes in a can, a frozen package or
a box is likely to have salt added as a preservative or flavor
enhancer.

Table salt and salty products can be easy to avoid, but it
is this "hidden salt" that often has consumers stumped. The
Food and Drug Administration (FDA) is now requiring
soft-drink manufacturers to list the sodium content of their
drinks on the bottles or cans. Many products are required to
list their sodium content, but be wary of their advertising
and labeling. Low sodium can mean different things for
different foods. For example, sodium-free drinks have to
contain less than five milligrams of salt per 12-ounce can.
"Very low sodium" will be less than 35 milligrams per can
and "low sodium" can be placed on cans containing 140
milligrams of salt or less according to the FDA's standards.

A typical slice of bread might contain over 200 milligrams of salt, a bowl of corn flakes over 300 milligrams, a
bowl of canned soup over 1,000 milligrams, a TV dinner
over 2,500 milligrams, a chicken dinner from a fast food
restaurant over 2,000 milligrams, and a large dill pickle over
1,000 milligrams

Studies of different nations around the world show that
high blood pressure is a problem only in societies where
people eat a lot of sodium, usually in the form of salt.
(Sodium, part of the sodium chloride salt molecule, is also
found in other forms. Technically, it is the sodium in salt
which is the villian in our fight against high blood pressure.
In this chapter, we will continue to use "salt" as a more
common term.)

High blood pressure rates are in direct proportion to the amount of salt consumed. The more salt that a particular society consumes, the greater the number of cases of severe high blood pressure. It is significant that the Greenland Eskimos and the Amazon Indians, who eat very little salt, have very little high blood pressure. But in the north of Japan, high blood pressure is common among the people whose diet contains large amounts of salt. Of course, in such societies other factors may also be at work, but the strong relationship between salt consumption and high blood pressure should be noted.

Perhaps you feel that you are just a "salt lover" because foods don't taste right to you without salt. But scientific studies indicate that salt preference is a learned habit — an acquired taste. As people reduce the amount of salt in their diets, they experience new flavor sensations that were masked by the large amounts of salt they used to eat. The true flavor of vegetables can be hidden by cooking with too much salt. In this sense, excessive salt can be a taste destroyer rather than a flavor enhancer.

One scientific study on salt consumption deals with twins. One twin was put on a low-salt diet. The other twin continued to consume a diet high in salt. After a few weeks, the twin on the low-salt diet learned to consume less salt and preferred to eat less salt. The other twin still was in the habit of consuming more salt and continued to prefer the high salt diet.

It will take about three months to lose the craving for salt, according to Mrs. Dash, a producer of no-salt products.

If you are concerned about giving up flavor in your

cooking, a little creativity can help add "spice" to your food while lowering the salt content. You do not have to sacrifice flavor when you cut down on sodium if you follow these suggestions from *Prevention* magazine and other authorities:

- Remove the salt shaker from your table.
- Never use salt in cooking or reduce your use of salt in recipes by at least one half.
- Use lemon juice on food instead of salt.
- Don't use onion or garlic salt as spices as they are just "flavored" salt. Use real onion or garlic for more flavor without the salt.
- When baking cakes, cookies, pies and puddings, use extracts instead of salt and reduce the sugar.
- Avoid store bought mixes for puddings, cakes, muffins, biscuits, cornbread, pancakes, etc. If you prepare your own from scratch you can control your ingredients.
- Read all labels to determine the sodium content and buy low-sodium products whenever possible. Watch for any additives that contain the word sodium, like sodium chloride, sodium hydroxide, monosodium glutamate (MSG), sodium bicarbonate, disodium phosphate, sodium benzoate, sodium propionate, sodium saccharin, disodium sulfite or others that contain salt like baking soda, baking powder and brine. Avoid these.
- Learn about the many natural herbs, spices, and fruit peels that are available. You may decide to

grow your own or to experiment with store-bought herbs.

- Use one of several salt-free mixtures of herbs and spices that are available for seasonings.

- Enjoy Mexican, Cajun, and Tex-Mex foods. The strong spices give flavor without adding salt. Beware of oriental food—it can be high in MSG which is high in salt.

- To spice chicken dishes, add fruit such as mandarin oranges or pineapples.

- Marinate chicken, fish, beef or poultry in orange juice or lemon juice. Add a homemade mustard or honey glaze.

- Marinate meat in wine or add wine to sauces or soups. If you thoroughly cook the dish, the alcohol will evaporate, but the flavor will be enhanced.

- Use fresh vegetables whenever possible. However, if you must used canned vegetables, wash them in cool water before using. Rinsing will help remove some of the salt added in the canning process.

- Just a little green pepper, parsley, paprika or red pepper can add a lot of flavor to a meal.

- Be sure to keep the meals attractive and include a variety of colors and textures. Most people are more tempted to add salt when the meal appears bland.

- Avoid taking sodium ascorbate, a formulation of vitamin C that contains sodium. If you need a vitamin C supplement while cutting back on sodium, ascorbic acid or calcium ascorbate forms of vitamin C are acceptable.

- Drink water with your meals and avoid soft drinks. Soft drinks are high in sugar, which dulls your taste buds and makes it more difficult to give up salt. Also, many carbonated drinks are high in salt content. Even some sugar-free soft drinks contain salt as sodium saccharin.

A test to show how much salt you are really consuming is available and may help some people monitor or reduce their sodium intake, says a study in *Archives of Internal Medicine* (144:1963-5). Thirty percent of people in the study had lower salt intake when they were using a chloride titrator strip at home. If you are not sure of your current salt intake or if you want to monitor your diet, check with your doctor about the titrator strip test.

Many scientific studies show that reducing salt intake will lower blood pressure in most people by a significant amount. Getting salt intake down into the range of 500 milligrams of salt per day helps the most. Reducing salt intake lowers blood pressure dramatically in some people because they have a hereditary tendency to hold on to salt or sodium. Thus, the benefits of reduced salt consumption are greatest for some of the people who need the benefits the most.

Certain people seem to be "salt retentive," and others are not as affected by salt, according to studies by Dr. L. K. Dahl in *Circulation Research* (40:1131-4). He found that some animals will develop high blood pressure, no matter how much salt they ingest. However, some people can consume large quantities of salt and never develop high blood pressure. Since there are not any tests to show who is salt retentive and who is not (although some are in the development stages), health professionals recommend that everyone reduce their salt intake as part of their high blood pressure treatment.

Diets low in fiber

Fiber supplements were given to people in one recent study, reported by Danish researchers in *The Lancet* (2,8559:622-3). The people in the study discovered that their systolic pressure (the upper number) dropped an average of 10 points, and the diastolic pressure dropped an average of five points in just three months. However, people in the study who took a placebo (a harmless, fake supplement) did not experience a change in their blood pressure.

Low-fiber diets have also been linked to heart and artery disease, constipation, appendicitis, diverticulosis, cancer of the large bowel, colon cancer, hemorrhoids and obesity.

One hundred years ago, the diet of the American and Canadian people contained an adequate amount of natural food fiber. Most bread was made with whole wheat flour which contained bran, the outer fibrous part of the wheat kernel. Coronary heart disease was rare at this time, and few people were troubled with appendicitis, diverticulosis, cancer of the large bowel, constipation, hemorrhoids, obesity or high blood pressure.

Then, in the last quarter of the 19th century, American industry made two discoveries which were hailed as breakthroughs. The first invention was the development of high-speed steel roller mills for flour milling. Food companies could produce a fine white flour which tasted better than most whole wheat flour and was less likely to spoil. The second development was the growth of the canning industry, and the canning process greatly reduced food fiber content.

These two changes took place over several years, and no one noticed that anything was wrong. But in the 20th century, scientists became puzzled at the persistent rise in certain death rates and obesity. Commentators noticed that people in less developed countries didn't suffer very much from these ills.

In the 1940s and 50s, Dr. Denis Burkitt, a British surgeon, noticed that he never found a case of diverticular disease or cancer of the colon in the thousands of rural tribesmen of East Africa that were autopsied. Further research showed that obesity, appendicitis, heart attacks, constipation and hemorrhoids were also extremely rare. Dr. Burkitt thought that the amount of fiber in the diet was the key. He, and other doctors like Cleave, Trowell and Heaton, investigated what happened to tribes who moved to African cities and adopted a typical, low-fiber western diet. The results confirmed the hypothesis. On a diet that had been depleted of bran and other fiber, many Africans became obese and developed all the other ills of western civilization, according to a report in the *Journal of the American Medical Association* (229:1068-74). Dr. Burkitt also linked high blood pressure with a lack of fiber in the diet (*JR College of Physicians*, 9:138-46).

Diets high in fat

Americans now consume almost 40 percent of their total calories from fat. High-fat diets along with other factors can cause hardening of the arteries which leads to higher and higher blood pressure over the years. Low-fat diets are associated with low blood pressure. Cutting fat intake levels in half can have a dramatic effect in reducing many cases of high blood pressure. A recent study by the U.S. Department of Agriculture found that eating less saturated fat could bring blood pressure down even in the absence of taking other beneficial measures. One researcher connected with the study said that it produced strong evidence that high-fat diets are undesirable because they lead to high blood pressure as well as other problems.

Educating yourself to identify and avoid high-fat foods, as well as increasing your fiber intake, are two of the most important steps you can take in changing to a healthier diet.

It is important to learn that all fats are not the same. Saturated fats raise the blood cholesterol and triglyceride levels. They are primarily found in animal and dairy products, such as fats in meats, egg yolks, milk, butter, cheese, cream and a few vegetable fats, such as coconut oil and hydrogenated vegetable shortening. Saturated fats are generally hard or solid at room temperature.

Replacing saturated fats with unsaturated fats, especially olive oil or fish oil may also help reduce high blood pressure. Remember, fats are present not only in meat and dairy products but also in fried foods, chips, creamed sauces, mayonnaise and pastries to name a few. Learn to read labels on cans and packages, looking for the fat content listed.

Polyunsaturated fats help to lower the levels of cholesterol in the blood and reduce the risk of high blood pressure. They are mostly derived from plant and vegetable sources, such as cottonseed, soybean, corn and safflower. Sunflower and sesame seeds, walnuts and pecans are also high in polyunsaturates. Polyunsaturated fats are usually soft or liquid at room temperature.

Monounsaturated fats, like olive oil, have been found to lower high blood pressure (*Journal of the American Medical Association*, 257:3251-56). At Stanford Medical School, Dr. Stephen Fortmann has found that one tablespoon of olive oil per day equalled a 3.1 drop in systolic (the upper number) pressure. If three tablespoons of olive oil or other monounsaturated fats were added to the daily diet or substituted for saturated fats, the systolic pressure could drop up to 9.4 points and the diastolic pressure could be reduced by 6.3 points, Fortmann claims. So increasing your monounsaturated fats while decreasing your saturated fats should help lower your blood pressure naturally.

Blood pressure drops significantly when the amount of fat is reduced to less than 40 percent of the diet, according to research by Dr. James M. Iacono of the U.S. Department of Agriculture. Use these tips to help reduce your cholesterol level and lower your blood pressure.

- Do not consume more than 100 milligrams of cholesterol for each 1,000 calories. Daily cholesterol should not exceed 300 milligrams.

- Saturated fats, found in red meats and dairy products, should be reduced to less than 10 percent of total calories. Foods that are rich in cholesterol should be avoided or drastically limited in the diet. These foods include: egg yolks, organ meats and most cheeses. Foods that should be reduced because they are high in saturated fats include: butter, bacon, beef, whole milk, cream, chocolate, almost any food of animal origin, hydrogenated vegetable shortening, coconut oil and palm oil.

- Unsaturated fats, such as fish and vegetable oils, may constitute as much as 10 percent of total calories.

- Total fat intake should be less than 30 percent of your daily calories.

- Try to avoid artificial and non-dairy creamers. If you need to use a powdered product (due to lack of refrigeration) use non-fat powdered milk. The instant, non-fat dry milk is convenient and has a lower fat content than a non-dairy cream substitute.

- Don't use foods containing coconut or palm oil. They are high in saturated fats.

- Cut back on beef, lamb and pork. Never eat any combination of them more than three times per week.

- Don't eat duck, goose or organ meats. They are high in fat content.

- If you must eat beef, use only lean cuts. When cooking at home, cut off all visible fat. Broiling, baking or roasting the meat in its own juices are the healthiest methods of preparation. When eating out, select the best quality cuts like a filet mignon or chateaubriand. Keep your portions small and don't use any gravy or sauce. Also, avoid casseroles and pot pies.

- When preparing chicken or turkey, be sure to cut off the skin because much of the fat is contained in the skin. Eat the light meat on a turkey or chicken because it contains less fat than the dark meat.
- When eating red meat, serve less meat by preparing dishes that use meat plus vegetables, pasta or grains. Then you can use less meat per person while still providing adequate protein, vitamins and minerals. Stir-frying strips of meat with vegetables or cooking them in a wok is a good example.
- For dishes that require hamburger, substitute ground turkey (without the skin) or, if you are a hunter, you may want to substitute ground venison.
- Don't buy meat, fish or poultry that is already breaded. If you want to bread the meat, make your own breading with plain bread crumbs, herbs, skim milk and egg whites. Don't deep-fry after breading.
- Avoid prepared luncheon meats. As well as being high in fat, they are high in sodium and nitrites. Sliced turkey breast, tuna salad and salmon salad (without mayonnaise) are good luncheon alternatives.
- When making soup, chili, or stew, place the broth in the refrigerator overnight. In the morning, remove any fat that has hardened at the top.
- Eliminate bacon bits from your diet. In salads and soups, try homemade croutons or herbs to add that "spicy" taste.
- Limit your egg yolks to two per week. This includes not only whole eggs, but eggs used in baking and cooking. To reduce cholesterol, *Cardiac Alert* (9:5) recommends using

two egg whites instead of one whole egg in cooking and baking.

- If you are using egg substitutes in trying to reduce your cholesterol intake, be careful. Many commercial egg substitutes are high in sodium or high in fat, even though they may be cholesterol-free. The American Heart Association recommends making a cholesterol-free egg substitute especially for use in baking: Beat three egg whites. Then add one-fourth cup non-fat milk, one tablespoon non-fat dry milk powder, and one teaspoon of polyunsaturated vegetable oil. Mix these four ingredients together to make a healthful egg substitute. According to an avid cholesterol-watcher, if you add a drop of yellow food coloring when making French toast, your family won't be able to tell the difference.
- Pre-packaged cake mixes, biscuits and pancake mixes are usually made with eggs. To make your own easy mix, combine all the necessary dry ingredients together and freeze. When you want to bake them, just take your mix out of the freezer and add the liquids. For the liquids, use only egg substitutes, non-fat milk and vegetable oils.
- When buying pasta, avoid noodles made with eggs.
- Avoid crackers that contain lard or "animal fat." Study the list of ingredients and buy only crackers made with acceptable vegetable oils. If a cracker leaves a grease stain on a paper towel, it contains too much fat.
- Avoid croissants.
- When buying bagels, choose those made with water rather than eggs.
- Switch from butter to margarine, preferably soft marga-

rine. People usually use less soft margarine because it is easier to spread, so it is the best choice.

- Don't use saturated fat like lard, shortening, or animal fat drippings for cooking. Use polyunsaturated oil like corn, safflower, sesame seed, cottonseed, soybean and sunflower oils. Monounsaturated oil like olive oil is best for your health, according to recent studies. Polyunsaturated oils are better for your heart and arteries than saturated fat, but not quite as good as monounsaturated oils.
- Eliminate one pie crust when baking pies. Make your pies "open-faced" rather than covering them with a second crust.
- In recipes, reduce the amount of added fat by one-third to one-half. Make up the difference by adding water. For example, if a recipe calls for one cup of oil, just add two-thirds cup of oil and one-third cup water. The next time you make the same recipe, try further reducing the amount of oil. Keep cutting back on the fat until you have reached the "lowest possible" fat level for that recipe.
- For sautéing, use a vegetable spray. The spray will limit the amount of fat you'll use in cooking.
- Avoid butter or sour cream on baked potatoes. Eating a plain baked potato is good for you and low in fat!
- Substitute low-fat cottage cheese or non-fat yogurt for sour cream in your favorite recipes.
- Avoid avocados and olives.
- Reduce the amount of peanut butter in your diet or eliminate it entirely.
- Eliminate potato chips, french fries and all fried "fast food" from your diet. When eating out, pull off all the

crisp, breaded portions from fried foods because they become saturated with cooking oil.

- Eliminating salt and butter or oil on popcorn is not always easy because without the liquid, it seems as if no other herbs or spices will stick to the popcorn. Try this delicious alternative. Lightly spray the popcorn with a "non-stick" vegetable spray, then add cinnamon, curry powder, onion powder (not onion salt), chili powder or other herbs for an enjoyable flavor without cholesterol or salt.

- If you want cheese, eat moderate amounts of the low-fat varieties like mozzarella, provolone and Swiss.
  For the taste of cheese, try a sprinkle of grated Parmesan cheese. It will still give you a cheese flavor but it contains fewer grams of fat.

- Avoid heavy salad dressings like blue cheese. Try to eat less salad dressing by placing the dressing on the side and using it only as necessary.

- Drink skim or low-fat milk. Avoid using whole milk; evaporated milk; or sweetened, condensed milk. If you want the convenience of condensed milk, use a low-fat evaporated milk powder. You also can buy evaporated skim milk in cans.

- Switch from ice cream to ice milk, sherbet, sorbet or frozen fruit treats. Beware of frozen yogurt, unless it is frozen low-fat yogurt.

- Limit your intake of baking chocolate or milk chocolate which contains highly saturated cocoa butter. Substitute cocoa powder for chocolate when possible in recipes. The American Heart Association recommends substituting three tablespoons cocoa powder and one tablespoon polyunsaturated oil for each one ounce piece of baking chocolate. It will cut the amount of saturated fat by over 60 percent.

- Try scallops. They are a low-fat and low-cholesterol seafood. Avoid lobster and shrimp.
- Avoid all foods prepared with sauces or gravies like a cheese sauce (described as "au gratin"), hollandaise sauce, lobster sauce, sweet and sour sauce, mayonnaise or regular gravy. Tomato sauce may also be high in salt!
- When buying processed foods, look for "catch words" on the label that indicate high fat or high cholesterol levels: lard, butter, shortening, fat, cream, hydrogenated or hardened oils, palm, palm kernel oil, coconut oil, whole-milk solids, whole-milk fat, egg solids, egg-yolk solids, suet, animal fat, animal by-products, cocoa butter, milk chocolate, or imitation milk chocolate. Avoid these products.
- Check food labels very carefully. Products labeled "low-cholesterol" may not conform to the same standards and could be high in saturated fats.
- Eat chick-peas, soybean products, oats, and carrots to help maintain low cholesterol levels. Oat bran is an excellent source of water-soluble fiber and can reduce blood cholesterol levels by 6 to 19 percent, based on data from the Lipid Research Clinic. Researchers at Northwestern University (*Journal of the American Dietetic Association*) discovered that about two cups of oatmeal or two oat bran muffins daily, combined with moderate levels of dietary fat and cholesterol, can lower cholesterol levels in just a few weeks. If you prefer oat bran muffins, be sure to use a low cholesterol substitute, rather than eggs, in the

muffins.

For best overall health, also eat foods like fruit, bran, whole grain breads and cereals. These foods may not lower cholesterol as well as oat bran does, but they are better than oat bran for preventing colon cancer and other diseases.

The role of vitamins and minerals in fighting high blood pressure

Protective potassium

There is evidence that potassium may help protect against high blood pressure. Part of the evidence, however, is clouded by the fact that societies which have high levels of salt consumption also have low levels of potassium consumption and vice versa.

A recent study at Duke University showed a significant drop in blood pressure in just two months when participants were given potassium. Although potassium lowered blood pressure in most individuals, blood pressure dropped the most in blacks. Potassium supplementation is extremely important in treating blood pressure problems in blacks, the doctors concluded in *Hypertension* (9:571-5).

Since this and other research indicates that supplemental potassium in the diet may help to lower blood pressure, it might be beneficial to eat more foods like bananas and citrus fruits, especially grapefruit, which are relatively high in potassium. Potassium is also widely distributed in foods

like cantaloupe, potatoes, raisins, pineapple juice, tomatoes, pears, apple juice, peaches, apples, meat, milk and
nuts.

People taking some diuretic drugs that reduce natural
potassium will also receive a prescription for a potassium
supplement.

Adults need 1,525 to 5,625 milligrams of potassium
daily, according to the U.S. Recommended Dietary Allowance. Potassium supplements should not be used by people
who have kidney disease or who are taking a prescription
diuretic that is potassium-sparing, because excessive potassium can be harmful or even fatal. Large doses of potassium
should be avoided unless prescribed by a doctor, because
high levels of potassium can cause heart attacks.

Additional calcium

Calcium supplements may help to lower some cases of
high blood pressure. According to new research published
in *Drug Therapy* (16,11:63), many people do not get enough
calcium. Inadequate calcium can lead to high blood pressure. Another study indicates that people with high blood
pressure consume 20 to 25 percent less calcium than people
who don't have high blood pressure. Signs of extremely
low levels of calcium in the diet are muscle cramps and
numbness in the limbs. Adequate vitamin D is necessary for
the absorption of calcium.

Dr. Lawrence Resnick at the New York Hospital-
Cornell Medical Center has found a link between people
who are salt retentive and calcium supplementation. The

more salt seems to affect someone's blood pressure, the more calcium supplements seem to improve their blood pressure, Resnick reports in the *Journal of Hypertension* (4:5182-5). Blacks and older people seem to benefit from calcium most, he says.

According to the *Journal of the American Medical Association* (257:1772-6), blood pressure dropped a "modest but significant" amount when men with normal blood pressure levels took 1,500 milligrams of calcium daily, according to research by Purdue University professor, Roseann Lyle, Ph.D.

Another study, by researchers from Johns Hopkins University School of Medicine, confirmed that the "degree to which blood pressure falls depends on the amount of calcium taken." Although blood pressure usually rises in the last trimester of pregnancy, blood pressure levels remained constant in women who received 1,500 milligrams of calcium per day (*Obstetrics and Gynecology*).

The risk of high blood pressure can be reduced by 22 percent in women who take 800 milligrams of calcium (the RDA) a day, reports a new study from Harvard Medical School. Blood pressure in women taking 800 milligrams per day was compared to women taking just 400 milligrams per day. Nutritionists have warned that most American women are not getting the RDA in their diets. They recommend either changing the diet by increasing low-fat dairy products, like skim milk, cottage cheese and yogurt, or taking daily calcium supplements.

Since taking calcium supplements or increasing the amount of calcium in the diet has few harmful side effects, extra calcium could be part of a blood pressure reducing therapy. Many people do not get the recommended daily allowance set by the U.S. government. So the supplements should not be "megadoses" but enough to meet our daily requirements. To avoid overdosing on calcium, increase the amount of calcium in the diet rather than relying on supplements. The RDA of calcium is 800 — 1,200 milligrams per day for adult males and females. Dairy products, salmon, sardines and leafy, green vegetables are the best natural sources of calcium.

Calcium supplementation should be avoided by people who have calcium oxalate kidney stones or by those with high blood-levels of calcium which make them more inclined to develop kidney stones.

Excessive amounts of calcium and vitamin D may make it difficult for the body to eliminate extra calcium, which can cause problems. Excessive vitamin D can be dangerous and actually can cause high blood pressure by promoting the formation of deposits in the arteries. The Recommended Dietary Allowance (RDA) of vitamin D is five micrograms per day for people over 50. It's double that for males and females from 11 to 24. Anyone under medical care should consult with his physician before greatly increasing vitamin D or calcium supplementation.

Even if you start taking supplemental calcium, do not stop taking blood pressure medication except on your doctor's advice.

Supplementing magnesium

A recent study by Dr. Burton M. Altura links low magnesium levels to high blood pressure. He believes that if the level of magnesium is too low, the calcium level becomes too high and the blood vessels contract, causing high blood pressure. In a separate study by Cornell University, Dr. Lawrence Resnick discovered that people with high blood pressure tend to have low magnesium in their red blood cells. Futhermore, Resnick claims that the patients who have their blood pressure under control have higher magnesium levels.

Another study in *The American Journal of Clinical Nutrition* (45:469-75) showed that older men who had the highest daily intake of magnesium had the lower blood pressure levels.

Other research shows that people have lower blood pressure if their water supplies have high concentrations of magnesium. Magnesium often is found with calcium in drinking water and in mineral supplements like dolomite.

Whole-grain products, vegetables, black-eyed peas, bananas, apples, peaches, lima beans, seafood and peanuts are good sources of magnesium. The water supply is also an excellent source of magnesium in many areas of the country where the water is relatively hard. Adult males need 350 milligrams of magnesium daily, while adult women need about 280 milligrams, according to the recommended daily allowance set by the U.S. government. Pregnant and nursing mothers need slightly more.

Increasing choline

Choline (a near-vitamin) supplements are reported to help control blood pressure. In a clinical study, one-third of a group of patients with high blood pressure had their blood pressure return to normal after receiving choline supplements. When the supplements were discontinued, their blood pressure rose once again. However, additional studies are needed to confirm that choline alone was responsible.

Lecithin, soybeans, eggs, fish, liver and wheat germ are rich natural sources of choline. Green vegetables, peanuts, brewer's yeast, and sunflower seeds are also good sources.

Excess vitamins

An overdose of vitamin D, from either excessive exposure to the sun, which acts on the skin to help produce vitamin D, or from taking high doses of vitamin D supplements, can lead to high blood pressure. Vitamin E, in doses larger than the RDA of eight to 10 milligrams per day, can also cause high blood pressure.

Cadmium cautions

Cadmium is a "heavy metal" which may be found in

trace amounts in water supplies in the United States and in other countries. The cause and effect relationship between high levels of cadmium and high blood pressure exists as it does with salt. In studies at Dartmouth Medical School (*American Journal of Physiology*, 214:469-74), Dr. Henry Schroeder found a direct link between cadmium and high blood pressure in rats. Cadmium is leeched into our water supply by soft water. Hard water does not seem to absorb cadmium as easily.

Your local water authority may be able to tell you if your water supply has higher than average concentrations of cadmium. If it does, using certified pure bottled water would be a good alternative.

Taking garlic

In studies at the University of Vienna, Dr. F.G. Piotrousky discovered that garlic reduced blood pressure in about 40 percent of his high blood pressure patients, reports *The Vitamin Bible*.

Other work at Loma Linda University in California has shown that four grams of garlic a day helped reduce blood fats in people with high cholesterol levels.

Researchers are not sure exactly why garlic lowers blood pressure and cholesterol. Eric Block, Ph.D., of the State University of New York at Albany, says the key to garlic's benefits is in its most active anti-clotting ingredient called ajoene.

Since garlic can cause bad breath and body odor, *The*

Vitamin Bible recommends taking it in perles (little time-release pills) that release in your intestines rather than your stomach. Researchers in Japan have produced another alternative called kyolic. *Prevention* magazine reports that kyolic provides the beneficial elements of garlic, is "odor-modified" and lowers blood fats without the odoriferous side effects.

Caffeine

Caffeine can raise blood pressure significantly and should be avoided. Caffeine consumption may create a false number of high blood pressure patients because caffeine raises borderline blood pressure levels, David Robertson, M.D. reported in *The New England Journal of Medicine* (298:181-186). Other studies in *The American Journal of Cardiology* (53:918-22) have found that systolic and diastolic blood pressure levels were raised an average of nine points with just two cups of coffee.

Caffeine is found in most "cola" and "pepper" drinks, some diet pills, coffee, tea and chocolate.

Black licorice

Black licorice or licorice extracts should be avoided if you suffer from high blood pressure, according to researchers at Tufts University. Black licorice can make the body hold on to salt, lose potassium and cause fluid retention (*The*

New England Journal of Medicine, 278:1381-3). People taking diuretics for their high blood pressure should be especially careful to avoid licorice because it seems to compound the problems and bad side effects of diuretic drugs. About 90 percent of the licorice imported into the United States is used in chewing tobacco. This is another reason people with high blood pressure should avoid all forms of tobacco.

Conclusion

The foods we eat and drink are such a major factor in causing high blood pressure that they can help us gain control over the disease rather than letting it control us. It takes knowledge and willpower to change our eating habits, but the payoff is far greater than any effort it takes to change. Not only will you feel better physically, but you will have the satisfaction that you have won the upper hand in your battle against high blood pressure if you take control of your diet.

CHAPTER 13

Breast Cancer

A dietary secret that might prevent breast cancer

Can you change your diet and prevent breast cancer? Some researchers are saying cautiously that such a dietary prevention plan might be good ammunition against one of the biggest killers of women. The secret — lower the amount of fat you eat, suggest two studies.

"Dietary fat is a risk factor for breast cancer," conclude researchers in an Israeli study of 2,300 women. In general, the Israeli study shows that women with high fat intakes are three times as likely to develop the types of tumors that turn into breast cancer. A high-fat diet promotes a change from benign (non-cancerous) breast disease to cancer, the researchers report in *The American Journal of Clinical Nutrition* (50,3:551). They point out that breast cancer develops in stages over a number of years, and if diet influences the process, women might be able to change their diet to help prevent cancer.

Diet apparently had no effect on two types of benign

breast disease. But, among those with the most advanced stage (grade 3) of benign breast disease, they spotted a link between high-fat diets and numbers of women with breast cancer.

"The results suggest that saturated fatty acids, but not the other food groups, are associated with grade 3 disease," according to the report. Although women with grade 3 disease ate more starches, sugars and proteins than other women, their fat intake was the greatest risk factor, the researchers conclude.

In a separate study published in the *Journal of the National Cancer Institute* (81:278-286), Dr. Paolo Toniolo of the Department of Environmental Medicine at New York University Medical Center studied over 700 Italian women by analyzing their daily diet in 70 food categories.

Most strongly linked to increased rates of breast cancer were dairy products like high-fat cheese and whole milk, he reports. Ranked just under dairy products were fats and meat. Women who ate foods rich in animal fat, such as meat and cured meat, showed a "modest" increase in the risk of breast cancer. "Consumption of fish, eggs, bread, pasta, olive oil, vegetables, and fruit did not reveal any evident relationship with breast cancer," the study says.

To reduce the risk of breast cancer, women need to reduce their consumption of total fat to less than 30 percent of their total daily calorie intake, saturated fat to less than 10 percent, and animal proteins to less than 6 percent, Toniolo suggests. The current typical American diet relies on fats for between 35 and 45 percent of total caloric intake.

Breast cancer develops from benign tumors. Although

numerous studies have shown that a high-fat diet influences the process, researchers are not sure how. They do know that breast-cancer patients in Japan have better outcomes than their counterparts in the U.S. One possible reason for the difference is that Japanese women generally eat a relatively low-fat diet. Obesity and low-fiber, low-carbohydrate diets may also contribute to lower survival rates, researchers speculate.

A high-fat diet also mightaffect the recovery rates of women who undergo breast cancer surgery, according to a related study in the *Journal of the National Cancer Institute* (81,16:1218). Swedish researchers evaluated the diets of 240 women aged 50 to 65 who had breast-cancer surgery between 1983 and 1986, says the *JNCI* report. They were particularly interested in protein, carbohydrate, fat, alcohol and vitamin intake, but they also considered other factors such as height, weight, smoking and physical activity.

Women with larger tumors reported eating less fiber, carbohydrates and vitamin A but more fat than women with smaller tumors. The high-fat eaters generally had larger tumors that spread further, the research indicates. Women who drank alcohol also showed an increased risk, researchers said.

This is also affirmed in a report in *Science News* (134:100) that says eating a lot of saturated fats makes active breast cancer grow faster and spread further, especially among older women. Canadian researchers studied the progress of recently diagnosed breast cancers in 666 women. Those with diets high in the kinds of fats found in butter, cheese, and coconut oil developed larger cancers that spread more rapidly to the lymph nodes, indicating a more severe (and less curable) form of the disease. The more cancer involves the lymph nodes, the harder it is to get rid of the disease.

On the other hand, those who ate foods high in polyunsaturated fats — such as corn, safflower, sunflower, and cottonseed oils — showed less invasion of the lymph tissues, the report said, indicating a more treatable form of the disease.

On the positive and preventive side, another study (reported in *Journal of the National Cancer Institute*, October 1988) showed that women who ate a "very low-fat diet" for a year developed fewer than half as many breast cancers as those who ate the "typical" diet. The low-fat diet apparently cut the cancer rate in half. Nearly 40 percent of the calories consumed in the "typical" American diet is in the form of fats, way too high for long-term health, the studies indicate.

According to the *JNCI* report, doctors at two Toronto hospitals put half of a group of 180 women whose mammograms showed unusual breast shadows on a specially formulated low-fat diet. Only about 20 percent of the diet's total calories was in the form of fat, while 56 percent was in carbohydrate form. The other half of the group, all of whom were diagnosed as facing higher risks of developing breast cancer, stuck to the "typical" diet—37 percent of its calories in fat and 43 percent in carbohydrates.

After a year, five on the "typical" diet developed breast cancer, but only two on the low-fat diet came down with the disease, the Toronto study showed. A larger, follow-up study is planned.

While many studies have demonstrated higher risks of

getting breast cancer because of fat-rich eating habits, the Canadian research is among the first to show that the growth and spread of the cancer is affected by what we eat — even after the cancer has become active!

This suggests that a low-fat diet could be an important weapon in fighting breast cancer, even after it has been diagnosed. The studies also hint that a low-fat diet over many months (1) could lower the risk of getting breast cancer; (2) could lessen the severity of the disease once it's active; and (3) could even increase the cure rate.

■ Reviewing 12 big studies about diet and breast cancer, researchers found a strong and consistent link between high-fat diets and increased breast cancer risks among women past menopause.

Eating fruits and vegetables, especially those high in vitamin C, definitely boosts protection against breast cancer, the same review says in the *Journal of the National Cancer Institute* (82,7:561).

■ Eating more fiber might protect against breast cancer, suggests a study reported in *The American Journal of Clinical Nutrition* (51,5:798).

Scientists studied 24 Seventh-Day Adventist women between the ages of 64 and 83, half of them vegetarians for more than a quarter-century. Other than what they ate, both groups were very similar.

The vegetarians ate more fiber than the other group and had significantly lower levels of estradiol and estrone, two hormones that have been linked to cancerous tumor growth.

Lower levels of these hormones may translate into lower cancer risks, the researchers speculate.

They think that steroid hormones stick to bran fiber, oat hulls, cellulose and lignin and are tossed out of the body quickly.

A high-fiber diet also might protect against endometrial cancers, the report says.

Other studies have shown similar links: eat more fiber and thus lower your risk of breast cancer, according to a review in *Nutrition and Cancer* (13,1:1).

■ If women in North America were to cut their daily consumption of saturated fats to less than one-tenth of their total calories, the breast cancer rate for women past menopause would drop 10 percent, says a report in *Science News* (137,16:245).

Just by eating enough fruits and vegetables to get 380 milligrams of vitamin C daily might drop the breast cancer rate by another 16 percent for all women over age 20, the report says.

That's more than six times the current officially Recommended Dietary Allowance of 60 milligrams. Check with your doctor before taking nutritional supplements.

Some other dietary strategies against this killer follow in detail in the following articles.

Eating fish might lower breast cancer risk

Women who eat fish regularly might lower their risk of

getting breast cancer, according to a preliminary statistical study in the journal *Nutrition and Cancer* (12,1:61).

Researchers at two Canadian cancer institutes analyzed how people eat in 32 countries around the world, including the United States. They looked at each country's average daily intake of total fats, animal fat, meat, cereal, milk, sugar, animal oil, total oils of all kinds, fish, coffee, tea, cocoa and riboflavin (one of the B vitamins). Then they compared peoples' diets with breast cancer rates for those countries.

They found what several other studies have shown — breast cancer rates go up where women eat more fats, especially animal fats. But the new study also indicated that in countries where fish consumption is high, breast cancer rates are lower.

The researchers linked this statistical finding with the possibility that diets with a lot of fish offer some protection against breast cancer. "The observation that percent calories from fish is inversely related to (breast cancer) risk implies a protective role for this dietary component," says the report.

They speculated that protection might come from the highly polyunsaturated omega-3 fatty acids contained in many kinds of fish from deep, cold waters.

They noted that very little research has been done before now to see if diets high in omega-3 fatty acids offer some protection against breast cancer. They called for more research to follow up their findings.

The same study also indicated that the rate of atherosclerosis (disease of the arteries caused by buildup of plaques containing fatty cholesterol) is linked in the same way. Where fish consumption (as a percent of total calories consumed) is high, artery disease is lower.

In the past several years, many studies have indicated the beneficial effect omega-3 (popularly known as fish oil) fatty acids have on lowering blood cholesterol levels, as well as a few problems with taking supplements.

For example, some people who take fish oil capsules experience burping and fishy aftertaste.

In addition, diabetics and people who are on blood-thinning medicines or aspirin therapy should avoid fish oil supplements unless they have specific permission from their doctor.

Studies are underway to determine omega-3's effect on several other kinds of cancer, as well.

In one case, omega-3 supplements given in capsule form seemed to help prevent the spread of cancer cells during and after cancer surgery, according to a Harvard Medical School study.

■ Eating more fish high in omega-3 fatty acids also might protect women against breast cancer because of its effect on female hormones.

Apparently, the omega-3 oils found in deep-water fatty fish help to cut levels of estradiol, a hormone that unfortunately promotes cancer growth.

The fish oil itself also seems to slow down tumor growth, reports a Rutgers University researcher in the *Journal of Internal Medicine Supplement* (225,731:197).

Despite a family history of breast cancer, women past the age of 60 have about the same risk as women with no such history, says a report in *Archives of Internal Medicine* (150,1:191).

The family history risk apparently affects mostly women of childbearing age.

The longer a woman lives without developing breast cancer, the less likely her heredity will catch up with her, at least in breast cancer risk, the study suggests.

Vitamin D 'unplugs' cancer cells

Investigators in England saw good results when they treated breast cancer cells in the laboratory with vitamin D three times a week.

More than 80 percent of all breast cancer tumors contain chemical "sockets" that plug in with the vitamin D, said the report in *The Lancet* (1, 8631:188).

Vitamin D in one form acts like a hormone in a woman's body, and attaches to hormonally-dependent tumors, they said.

Once attached to a tumor, the vitamin D acts to halt the spread of cancer cells and works to return cell activity to normal, the report said.

Broccoli and brussels sprouts might help prevent breast cancer

You might prevent breast cancer by eating more cabbage, broccoli and other cruciferous vegetables, suggests a new study published in the *Journal of the National Cancer Institute* (82,11:947).

Scientists are excited about the potential of a powerful cancer-fighting substance discovered in these vegetables.

The substance — indole-3-carbinol — seems to convert one cancer-promoting form of the female sex hormone estrogen into a harmless form.

That harmless form also might block absorption of the "bad" kind of estrogen by breast cells, suggests a report of the study in *Science News* (137,24:375).

The active forms of estrogen have been blamed by many scientists for triggering breast cancer growth.

Anything that blocks active estrogen from breast cells could prevent the formation of cancerous growths, says the *SN* report.

Scientists fed volunteers 500 milligrams of indole-3-carbinol daily for a week.

They used a manufactured form of the natural chemical.

The daily dose was the equivalent of eating about half a head of cabbage a day.

The production of estrogen-blocker jumped by 50 percent after just one week, the study shows.

The results might explain why Asian women—who eat a lot of cruciferous vegetables — have much lower breast cancer rates than American women.

The problem is one of taste — many people just don't like to eat their veggies, especially broccoli and brussels sprouts.

Dr. Jon J. Michnovicz, one of the researchers who found the cancer fighter, suggests that indole-3-carbinol could be produced in a pill form.

That would allow women who don't like cabbage to take a daily supplement to prevent breast cancer, suggests the report in *SN*.

No such supplement currently exists.

Vegetables containing indole-3-carbinol include cabbage, broccoli, Brussels sprouts, mustard greens, bok choy, kale, collards, turnip greens and cauliflower.

All these are members of the cruciferous family of vegetables.

The flowers of these vegetables resemble small crosses. Their Latin name means "cross-like."

Several studies have shown that eating a lot of vegetables protects against several other forms of cancer, notably colon and rectal cancers.

But researchers until now had thought the protection came from the fiber contained in the vegetables.

This is the first study to show that a specific natural chemical may be responsible for at least part of the protective effect against breast cancer.

One of every 10 American women will eventually develop breast cancer, according to government statistics.

Slightly more than seven out of 10 women are still living five years after being diagnosed as having breast cancer. Those survival rates have remained about the same for more than 25 years.

Indulging a sweet tooth might increase your risk of breast cancer

A taste for sweet things might be dangerous for women with diagnosed breast cancer, suggest two scientific studies.

Eating and drinking foods with high-sugar contents produced faster-growing and more deadly tumors in animal tests, report cancer researchers in *Clinical Nutrition* (9,2:62).

Mice fed diets that were high in sugar were nearly three times more likely to die quickly than mice on low-sugar diets, the report says.

Tumors seemed to thrive on sugary diets and were nearly five times as deadly as the same kind of cancerous tumors in mice on a low-sugar diet, reports the journal article.

The researchers found that adding vitamin E and selenium to the diets helped a little bit.

Mice on high-sugar diets that received the two nutrients — known as antioxidants — still developed big, fast-growing tumors, but the tumors were less deadly.

Antioxidants like vitamin E act like scavengers in the blood, neutralizing cancer-promoting chemicals known as oxidants.

The researchers speculate that sugary diets trigger lots of insulin production by the body. Insulin is needed to help body cells use the right amount of sugar.

But insulin also acts like a powerful fertilizer to tumor cells, greatly speeding up the growth of the harmful cells.

The more insulin the body produces in response to a sugary diet, the more fertilizer is poured on cancer cells, the report suggests.

Backing up the suspicions about sugar, a statistical study in the same issue of *Clinical Nutrition* documents a strong link between sugar eating and breast cancer deaths.

Some of the same researchers checked records of average sugar consumption in 20 countries around the world.

Then they cross-checked rates of breast cancer and deaths from breast cancer in those same countries for women between the ages of 55 and 74.

Sure enough, countries with the lowest sugar consumption per person — like Japan and Hong Kong — also have the lowest rates of death from breast cancer, the report says.

Those countries with the biggest hunger for sugar — like the United States and Great Britain — have the highest rates of breast cancer deaths.

The average person in the United States takes in two pounds of sugar a week, the report says.

But the average Japanese citizen eats less than half that much sugar in a week — 14 ounces on average, the report says.

The report notes that the death rate from breast cancer in Japan is about one-fifth that of the United States.

The statistical comparison took into account and adjusted for other factors, including average daily fat intake, the journal article says.

Underlying both reports is the suggestion that slower-growing tumors result in people living longer after diagnosis of breast cancer.

Based on their findings, the researchers suggest that women with diagnosed breast cancer should cut back on sweets and maintain a low-sugar diet.

Soybeans and breast cancer

Would eating soybeans several times a week slash your risk of getting breast cancer?

Some researchers suspect that a diet loaded with soybeans may be the reason Asian women have one-fifth the number of cases of breast cancer that American women have, says a report in *The Atlanta Journal* (108,22).

Women of the East eat tofu, or soybean curd, the way we Americans eat eggs and potatoes.

So far, animal tests have raised hopes that soybeans may provide some powerful cancer prevention, but no tests have been made on people.

Soybeans contain isoflavones, substances that may block some cancer-causing chemicals. The big drawback — soybean products like tofu generally don't win any taste tests.

Fresh fruits and vegetables help prevent cancer

Eating a lot of fresh fruits and vegetables may help you prevent cancer, researchers report in *Food, Nutrition and Health* (13,9: 2).

Fruits and vegetables contain small amounts of acids

called phenols, which stop cancer-causing agents from attacking healthy cells.

Where can you find phenols? In almost all fruits and vegetables, but potatoes, grapes and nuts have especially high amounts.

Because phenols are surprisingly plentiful in the diet, scientists say that some people may take in more than one gram every day (although they haven't yet determined the ideal amount).

To get the anticancer benefits, you must eat fresh fruits and vegetables, because processing vegetables and storing them destroy phenols.

Scientists are now looking for ways to "fortify" fruits and vegetables with phenols in the laboratory.

CHAPTER 14

Cancer

Preventing cancer: Your diet can make the difference

Despite ever-increasing evidence that what we eat can play a major role in preventing many forms of cancer, only about one in five Americans regularly eats the right kinds of foods to get the highest protection.

Researchers at the National Cancer Institute in Bethesda, Md. surveyed 11,658 white and black adults about a typical day's diet. The study showed that only 16 percent of those surveyed ate high-fiber cereals or whole-grain breads. Only 18 percent ate at least one green vegetable (high in cancer-fighting beta carotene), and only 20 percent had any kind of fibrous vegetables. High vitamin-C fruits and vegetables came out a little better (28 percent).

On the other hand, 55 percent of all adults ate red meat, rich in cholesterol, at least once a day. Breakfast and processed lunch meats, high in many suspected cancer-causing preservatives, appeared on the menus of 49 percent of the males and 37 percent of the females surveyed.

The large study showed, in fact, that many of us tend to eat just those things that are worst for our health and avoid those foods that are best for us.

Income levels and where we live make a difference, the study showed. Southerners balanced a plus with a minus, eating the least red meat but ignoring high-fiber cereals. Young white males seem to avoid foods that are good sources of vitamins A and C. The higher the income, the more red meat, produce and high-fiber cereals are consumed.

Numerous scientific studies advise us to eat fruits and vegetables, whole grains and foods rich in vitamins A and C and fiber, and to do it every day. The same studies say we should cut way down on red meats and fat and avoid any foods that have been salt-cured, nitrite-cured, smoked or pickled.

On the same lines, a report in *The American Journal of Clinical Nutrition* outlines how your diet can mean the difference between healthy maturity and lingering illnesses.

Here's a sampling from that issue (49,5:993):

About 35 percent of all cancers currently are linked to poor diet, according to the report. A high-fiber diet has been shown to reduce colon-cancer risk, and a high-fat diet increases breast-cancer risk. The experts have devised "interim" dietary guidelines, which include a varied, well-balanced diet (fruits, vegetables, whole grains) with reduced fat, salt, alcohol and processed foods.

You should also watch your weight.

Cancer Prevention Tips

- Avoid drinking or cooking with chlorinated water
- Avoid using talcum powder in the genital areas
- Avoid drinking coffee, either regular or decaffeinated
- Avoid contact with asbestos
- Avoid excessive exposure to the sun
- Avoid fried foods
- Avoid processed foods containing carcinogenic additives
- Avoid barrier forms of contraception
- Eat foods rich in vitamin D, calcium, molybdenum, and selenium, such as fish, whole-grain foods, wheat germ, and beans
- Include lysine, an amino acid, in your diet
- Eat crunchy, yellow and dark-green, leafy vegetables
- Reduce sodium and increase potassium in your diet
- Eat foods rich in dietary fiber
- Avoid cigarettes
- Avoid excessive amounts of alcohol

(**Source** — *Natural Health and Wellness Encyclopedia, FC&A Publishing,* 1988)

Cervical cancer

Vitamins that might fight cervical cancer

Women with abnormal cervical cells sometimes have low blood levels of vitamin A, vitamin C, and folic acid, one of the B vitamins. These abnormal cells, known as cervical dysplasia, can develop into cancer of the cervix in women. The cervix is the opening to the womb.

Research is now underway at Albert Einstein College of Medicine in New York to see if adding these vitamins to the diet can help reverse the abnormal cell development and help prevent cervical cancer.

Other studies have linked low levels of vitamin A to development of cervical cancer (*Gynecology and Oncology*, 30,2:187 and *American Journal of Obstetrics and Gynecology*, 148,3:309). But this new research will focus on the role of vitamin supplements in preventing cervical cancer.

Colon, intestinal and rectal cancer

High-fiber diet slashes rectal cancer rates

A high-fiber diet can slash your risk of rectal cancer, a four-year scientific study indicates. It can do this by reducing the number of non-cancerous tumors of the rectum, according to encouraging results reported in the *Journal of the National Cancer Institute* (81,17:1290).

What you eat is important because colon cancer is the second deadliest cancer in the U.S, and each year, 145,000 new cases are diagnosed.

In 1987 alone, colon cancer killed 60,000 Americans.

Most of its victims are middle-aged or beyond.

The disease can be controlled and even cured if caught in its early stages.

Best results seemed to happen with dietary fiber levels of nearly one ounce every day. That's about twice what most Americans eat regularly. The high-fiber diet seems to fight formation of benign rectal polyps. These are little tumors on stalks. Sometimes polyps look like tiny mushrooms growing out of the walls of the rectum and lower intestine.

These benign polyps, if not discovered or if left untreated, almost always turn into cancer, the report says. Previous studies have shown that high-fiber diets decrease risks of getting colon cancer. So researchers studied 58 people to determine whether they would reap the same benefits farther down the digestive tract.

Before the study began, patients were given a baseline examination to calculate the size and number of polyps. There were three groups: sixteen took vitamin C and vitamin E with a low-fiber supplement (vitamin group), twenty were given the vitamins with a high-fiber supplement (high-fiber group), and 22 received only a low-fiber breakfast cereal supplement (control group).

On the average, the vitamin group took in 11.3 grams of wheat fiber per day; the high-fiber group, 22.4 grams; and the control group, 12.2 grams. One ounce equals just over 28 grams. Researchers chose wheat fiber and vitamins C and E because they have shown the best results in anticancer studies. The wheat fiber — a non-water-soluble kind of dietary fiber — came from a common brand of breakfast cereal.

Every three months, researchers examined all the groups to see if the number of tumors rose or fell. In addition, nurses counseled people having trouble following the diet. After six months, polyp size and numbers had been cut in half in the high-fiber group, researchers said. Those who took vitamins with a low-fiber cereal generally broke even — no increase and no decrease in tumors.

"A high prescribed fiber intake and, to a lesser extent, a high vitamin intake, were associated with lower polyp number ratios," according to the report. This is good news, especially for people with a family history of rectal tumors.

Compliance in the study was low, meaning that the people being studied failed to stick strictly to their diets. That surprised the researchers, since the patients were aware of their cancer risk. Compliance was highest overall for the high-fiber group, which also showed the best results, followed by the vitamin group and the control group.

In addition to diet therapy, treating polyps in the colon with nonsteroidal anti-inflammatory drugs (NSAIDs) shows promising results, according to *Medical World News* (30,18:23). NSAIDs are effective because they limit the production of prostaglandins, a type of fatty acid, high concentrations of which are found in tumors.

Taken daily, a NSAID called indomethacin stopped polyp formation in 11 patients who had already undergone surgery to remove colon tumors. More studies are planned.

Fruit fiber enters the fray

The results of a study by researchers from the University of Utah School of Medicine say, "Of the food groups examined, fruit appeared to have the greatest protective effect. High intakes of fruits and vegetables had a beneficial effect on the colon."

Other studies (*Journal of the National Cancer Institute* 55:15-18 and *Journal of Epidemiology* 109:132) have shown a direct link between high fiber and a lower incidence of colon cancer. Despite those findings, doctors were not sure what type of fiber was most effective.

For this study, the Utah team evaluated "various types and sources of fiber in the diet" of more than 500 men and women for five years. Crude fiber was the most important fiber-type in the study, as it consistently decreased the risk of colon cancer in both men and women.

The average person consumes "only 15 to 20 grams of fiber a day, when they need 25 to 40 grams," according to Dr. Denis Burkitt, one of the most respected researchers in the field of dietary fiber.

By increasing daily intake of soluble fiber and insoluble fiber to at least 25 grams, adults and children can help prevent colon cancer as well as "digestive disorders such as constipation, irritable bowel syndrome (IBS), hemorrhoids, and diverticular disease," Dr. Burkitt said.

Soluble fiber, like pectin in apples, is easily dissolved in water. Soluble fiber bonds chemically with certain substances like cholesterol and moves them quickly through the digestive tract.

Insoluble fiber, like cellulose (in whole grains) and hemicellulose (in vegetables) doesn't dissolve in water. Instead such fiber absorbs water like a sponge, softening waste products in the intestines and speeding it out of the body.

Both kinds of fiber are needed for healthy digestion.

Put the starch back into the diet

Years ago, starch was something other than what you spray on shirts to be ironed.

Starches were considered a distinct food group, and youngsters were encouraged to eat something from that group two or three times a day to ensure a healthy diet.

Come the Nineties, and starches are now "complex carbohydrates."

Despite the trendy name, starchy foods are still the same ones we knew as children: potatoes and rice and breads and foods made from grains.

One British researcher believes that starchy foods may be what's missing in our search for foods that protect from cancers of the colon and rectum.

No, it's not the fiber in those foods, either, although fiber certainly is beneficial.

Instead, believes K.W. Heaton of the Bristol Royal Infirmary in England, it's the starchy foods that "escape" digestion in the stomach and small intestine that might do us the most good.

Those "escaped" starches are quickly fermented in the large intestine (colon) and pass quickly on through the bowel.

The fermentation and quick passage seem to protect the colon from harmful substances in foods.

One clue supporting this theory is the finding that people who develop a lot of precancerous growths in their colons also seem to be unusually efficient at digesting starch before it gets to the colon, says Heaton.

Even those people could help themselves by eating starchy foods in less-digestible forms, the researcher suggests.

For example, instead of using baked flour products, eat a lot of whole grains like rice.

Take these veggies

President Bush might not like broccoli, but your colon does! According to *Nutrition and Cancer* (13,4:271), "vegetable fibers may generally be more protective against colorectal carcinogenesis (cancer) than cereals."

That's because vegetables are more "fermentable" than cereal fibers.

Fermentation refers to one of the processes in which the body (particularly the stomach and intestines) breaks down foods into usable compounds necessary for proper nutrition.

A fiber source that is highly fermentable appears to be a strong warrior against cancer.

Fermentation takes place when the "good" bacteria in

the intestines break down vegetable or animal matter.

During that process, nutrients are released into the intestines. This process supplies the body with important nutrients.

And, equally important, fermentation helps resupply the intestinal bacteria with vital nutrients.

The bacteria help keep the bowel healthy and functioning properly and help protect the colon from cancer.

The *Nutrition and Cancer* report indicates that vegetable and cereal fibers release a continuous stream of nutrients, unlike some starches and sugars.

Carbohydrates from starches and sugars break down rapidly and might actually increase the risk of colorectal cancer, the report says.

With a garden of varieties to choose from, vegetables sprout up as a healthy alternative for your fight against colon cancer.

Constipation dangers

Not only is constipation and a slow bowel uncomfortable, at times, it may actually lead to the buildup of cancer-causing chemicals.

Diet plays an important role in preventing this unhealthy build-up. A British study looked at the diets of 50 patients with colon cancer and the diets of non-cancer patients.

The researchers' conclusion? A lack of fiber in the diet predisposed the patients to their cancers.

The mechanism of the connection between fiber and

cancer prevention is not entirely clear.

Many believe that the slow movement of food through the intestines leads to the production of cancer-causing chemicals by undesirable bacteria that thrive in the environment of a constipated colon.

The slow movement of the fecal mass keeps these irritants in contact with the colon for a long time.

What's in the fiber

Scientists have discovered an active ingredient in dietary fiber that may help to prevent cancer and treat established cancer. According to the journal *Carcinogenesis* (10,3:625), fiber contains inositol hexaphosphate (InsP6), which was effective in significantly reducing the size and number of colon and rectal cancers in rats and mice.

Inositol hexaphosphate, also known as phytic acid, is found in wheat, corn, oats and rice. It is "an abundant plant seed component present in many, but not all, fiber-rich diets," researchers report in the journal *Cancer* (56,4:717). Until now, doctors knew that dietary fiber helps reduce the risk of cancer, but they believed it was because fiber helps move waste through the body and reduces the amount of time that cancer-causing substances can build up in the colon.

In a recent study, Dr. Abulkalam Shamsuddin of the University of Maryland in Baltimore removed InsP6 from fiber and gave it to test animals in their drinking water. The test animals otherwise had no extra fiber in their diet. Even without the roughage, "the treated animals developed significantly fewer cancers, and 'their cancers were two-thirds smaller' than those of untreated controls," Dr. Shamsuddin said.

In an earlier study reported in *Carcinogenesis* (9,4:577), he found that inositol hexaphosphate reduced the effects of cancer in the large intestine. Other studies by Graf and Eaton reported in *Cancer* (56,4:717) also showed that InsP6 suppresses colon cancer and other inflammatory bowel diseases.

Shamsuddin decided to study the effects of InsP6 when he noticed that groups with high-fiber diets often had different rates of cancer. The amount of InsP6 in the diet seemed to be the only difference, so he decided to test InsP6's effectiveness without the fiber content.

Since InsP6 and Ins are effective agents against large intestinal cancer "in two different species with two different carcinogens (cancer-causing agents), are found naturally, and have relatively little toxicity, they should therefore be seriously considered in our strategies for prevention" of this cancer in humans, Dr. Shamsuddin reported to the Eighth Annual Meeting of the American Association for Cancer Research. Tablets or capsules of InsP6 could one day be used in the treatment of human cancer because InsP6 can be extracted easily, he said.

Research by Dr. Lillian Thompson at the University of Toronto has also shown that InsP6 has an anti-cancer effect in mice. Other studies showed that InsP6 given after five months of cancer helped to slow the cancer growth.

Common bean and pea have secret weapon

It's no longer a secret — the food on your dinner plate can greatly influence your health. In fact, if you choose your menu wisely, you can actually build a line of defense against cancer.

The common bean and pea are two kinds of those cancer-fighting foods, reports *Nutrition and Cancer* (14,2:85). In a recent study, those people who frequently ate legumes (beans, peas, lentils, soybeans, etc.) cut their risk of colon and rectal cancer in half.

The secret behind the anti-cancer effects of legumes is a substance known as protease inhibitor (PI). Protease inhibitor is a strong anti-cancer ingredient, and legumes contain high concentrations of this cancer-fighting substance.

Another plus: adding more foods with a high PI content to your diet helps protect you from colon and rectal cancer without causing any adverse side effects.

Legumes are inexpensive and tasty. Add this to their new-found reputation as a serious cancer fighter and you have every reason to say, "Pass the peas, please!"

What's left after the fiber

In addition to crude fiber, fruits and vegetables, another natural ingredient — ash — seems to provide protection against colon cancer, according to a new study in the *Journal of the National Cancer Institute* (80,18:1474). Ash is defined as "the mineral residue after all the combustible (burnable) components of food samples have been removed."

Calcium, which is a major component of ash, was also found "to have a strong dose-response protective effect against colon cancer." That means the protective effect went up as the dose went up.

Antacid stops 75% of colon cancers?

Taking twice the current Recommended Dietary Allowance (RDA) of calcium every day might prevent nearly 75 percent of all colon cancers, says a cancer researcher in *Medical World News* (31,4:22).

That's equal to about eight regular non-prescription calcium carbonate antacid tablets.

Evidence of calcium's prevention power is snowballing, with 60 studies worldwide now reporting the mineral's natural benefits.

In light of these encouraging study results, some researchers are suggesting a change in the RDA of calcium for adults.

Currently, the RDA for people over 50 is 800 milligrams a day.

It takes 1,200 milligrams of calcium a day to prevent colon cancer in people under the age of 49, some pro-calcium researchers say.

People over age 49 need 1,500 milligrams daily to get the prevention effect, they suggest.

Check with your doctor before taking supplements of any kind, and especially before taking more than the RDA.

Researchers really don't know how calcium works, but some believe it fights the effects of a high-fat diet on the colon wall, according to a report in *Preventive Medicine* (18,5:672).

Studies have shown that fatty foods speed up cell growth in the colon, and such spurts are the first step to tumor development.

Calcium travels throughout the digestive tract, working to keep cell growth under control.

It gets there by way of vitamin D — a rapid transit system of sorts — which transports energized calcium to the intestines, primed for preventing bad cell growth.

Although the experts agree that calcium does help fight colon cancer (and other diseases), they disagree on which form of calcium is best. Would a natural form of calcium be best?

Excellent natural sources of vitamin D are sunshine, tuna, fish liver oils and fortified milk.

You also can buy calcium supplements over-the-counter, meaning you don't need a doctor's prescription.

Taking eight carbonate tablets (such as Tums) a day would provide about 1,600 milligrams of calcium. (One regular Tums contains about 200 milligrams of calcium.)

If you take calcium supplements, you should drink at least two liters of fluid every day, recommends Dr. Cedric Garland, a professor at the University of California at San Diego.

Too much calcium and not enough fluids could add up to a case of painful kidney stones.

You shouldn't take more than 16 calcium carbonate tablets in a day nor for longer than two weeks.

Check with your doctor before taking antacids or any supplements.

Milk: a mixed blessing

Mother was partly right when she told you to drink your milk.

Just two eight-ounce glasses of fortified milk a day provide enough calcium and vitamin D to help lower your colon-cancer risk, according to *Medical World News* (31,1:41).

In a recent study, seven men at high risk for colon cancer took 1,250 milligrams of calcium every day for one week. In four men, extra calcium cut the amount of a cancer-causing enzyme in the colon by 50 percent.

This finding confirms several previous studies.

Researchers also found that people with higher levels of vitamin D — at least 20 milligrams per milliliter of blood serum — had a 70 percent decrease in colon-cancer risk compared to people with lower vitamin D levels (lower than 20 milligrams/ml).

Even so, the saturated fats in dairy products make milk a mixed blessing. For the cautions needed, see the following stories.

Drink low-fat milk instead

Could the kind of milk you drink increase your risk of getting cancer? Researchers in Buffalo, N.Y. think that it could.

According to a report in *Nutrition and Cancer* (13,1&2:89), researchers at Roswell Park Memorial Institute compared the risks of drinking whole milk and the risks of drinking fat-reduced milk (2 percent or skim milk) and found some surprising results.

Their findings show that the fat content of milk is a large risk factor.

Drinking milk with the highest fat content increases cancer risks. Drinking fat-reduced milk appears to protect against many of the same risks.

The study suggested that those who drank large amounts of whole milk were more likely to have cancer than those who never drank whole milk.

And there were fewer cases of cancer among the patients who drank large amounts of fat-reduced milk than among the patients who did not drink fat-reduced milk.

These findings suggest that drinking whole milk may cause cancer, whereas drinking fat-reduced milk may actually help prevent cancer.

Whole milk and fat-reduced milk are both rich sources of calcium, riboflavin, vitamin A and vitamin C.

However, whole milk is the fourth-largest source of calories and the second-largest source of saturated fats in the typical American diet.

Whole milk is also a large source of cholesterol.

Researchers suggest that drinking fat-reduced milk offers all the nutritional benefits found in whole milk without adding the additional fat, calories, and cholesterol from whole milk.

Your best bet: drink fat-reduced milk.

It provides you with vital nutrients without extra fats and cholesterol and helps protect you from the cancer risks that seem to be linked to whole milk.

However, some women should stay away from milk and related dairy products altogether. See the article about ovarian cancer in this chapter.

Sitting on the risk

If you sit down to a meal of cheese steak very often, your colon may be paying a high, even deadly, price.

Those two actions — sitting a lot and consuming a lot of fatty meats and dairy products — are the very highest risk factors for developing colon and rectal cancers, says a major new study in the *Journal of the National Cancer Institute* (82,11:915).

The study of hundreds of Chinese in America and in China itself pointed at two main villains: saturated fat and a sedentary lifestyle.

In fact, the study found that your cancer risk increases as you spend more time sitting.

Eating more than 10 grams a day of saturated fat, along with physical inactivity, "could account for 60 percent of colon and rectal cancer incidence among Chinese-American men and 40 percent among Chinese-American women," the report says.

Ten grams is slightly more than one-third of one ounce.

Researchers compared the two groups because they wanted to find out why colon and rectal cancer rates are four to seven times higher among Chinese who move to America than rates among the general population in mainland China itself.

They took into account the difference in diets in the two countries.

For example, a typical mainland Chinese person will eat more calories per day than his Chinese-American cousin.

But more of those native-country calories will come from carbohydrates and starches.

In China, the average person will get about 54 percent of his protein requirements from grains like rice, and only 20 percent from meat (mainly pork) and fish, the report says.

Over here, however, the Chinese-American will reverse that—60 percent of his protein from meat and fish, and only 17 percent from rice and other grains.

Both groups got about four to five grams a day of crude fiber.

Chinese-Americans took in more daily calcium and beta-carotene, a forerunner of vitamin A.

In this study, the two nutrients plus fiber seemed to give some protection against the two bowel cancers.

After accounting for diet differences, the two culprits of saturated fat and sedentary lifestyle stood out in the lineup as the major risk factors for developing colon and rectal cancer, this country's second-leading cancer killer.

Interestingly enough, people living in two mainland Chinese cities also had higher cancer rates, suggesting that city diets might not be as healthy as country diets.

Saturated fat is the stuff that makes butter and animal fat solid at room temperature.

Vegetable fats, on the other hand, usually contain monounsaturated and polyunsaturated fats and are generally liquid at room temperature.

Vegetable fats like corn oil and soybean oil make up most of the liquid cooking oils these days.

Nutritionists recommend that you eat foods low in saturated fats.

They suggest that you try to get less than a third of your daily calories from fats of all kinds, and less than one-tenth of your total calories from saturated fats.

Potassium protector

Some scientists have suspected that higher levels of the mineral nutrient potassium might help protect you against intestinal cancers.

Now an animal study suggests that such protection might be determined by the ratio of potassium to sodium in the body.

The higher the potassium-to-sodium ratio, the better, indicates a study in *Nutrition and Cancer* (14,2:95).

Researchers found that rats with four times as much potassium as sodium in their supplemented diets had one-eighth the number of intestinal tumors.

That was when compared with the ones fed a diet containing a potassium-sodium ratio of two-to-one, the report says.

Nutritionists recommend that you get at least 1,600 to 2,000 milligrams per day of potassium in your diet. That's not hard if you eat a lot of unprocessed fruits and vegetables and fresh meat.

Taking in more potassium than sodium also helps keep your blood pressure under control.

Getting too much potassium can be as bad as getting too

little. A daily intake of around 18 grams (that's 18,000 milligrams) can cause serious heart disturbances, even cardiac arrest.

Check with your doctor before taking potassium or any kind of dietary supplements.

Salty diet linked to colorectal cancer

Australian researchers say people who eat an ounce or more of salt a week face higher risks of getting colon and rectal cancers. The risk is greater for men than for women, says the report in *Nutrition and Cancer* (12,4:351). The same study also found that getting more potassium, particularly from fruits and vegetables, seems to protect men and women from both kinds of cancers.

Leukemia

Severe form of leukemia halted with vitamin A drug

French researchers report promising results in treating a severe kind of blood cancer with a concentrated form of vitamin A. Using retinoic acid, a derivative of vitamin A, three out of four people with acute myeloid leukemia were disease-free up to nine months after treatment stopped, according to a report in *The Lancet* (2,8665:746).

Lung cancer

This nutrient helps prevent lung cancer

For generations children have been encouraged, cajoled and forced by their parents to eat carrots because of the supposed benefits to the eyes. Research now suggests that the vitamin A found in carrots does a lot more than enhance eyesight: it may help prevent lung cancer.

A study at the State University of New York at Buffalo compared the diets of 900 healthy people with that of 450 lung cancer patients. Researchers found that those with lung cancer ingested much less beta-carotene than the healthy people, according to *Prevention* magazine.

Beta-carotene, found in large quantities in carrots, is converted by the body to vitamin A. Vitamin A helps maintain the epithelial tissue that lines part of the lungs. It is thought either beta-carotene directly "protects the lungs from cancer," *Prevention* says, or that "vitamin A squelches free radicals." (Free radicals are the compounds in the body which are thought to trigger cancer).

The difference between the beta-carotene intake of those with high and low risks of cancer "amounted to about 6,750 international units (IU), the amount provided by a single carrot," *Prevention* reports.

Oral cancer

Raw fruit lowers oral cancer risk

Cancer of the mouth is a devastating, disfiguring disease thought by many researchers to be linked to smoking, especially pipes, and use of chewing tobacco and snuff. It usually starts as a red or thickened white patch or a painless ulcer inside the mouth. The abnormal area, known as a lesion, is most common on the lips, tongue and floor of the mouth.

Cancer of the mouth and throat ranks number six on the most-common-cancer list among men and women combined. But men over 45 are twice as likely as women to develop it. Some forms of oral cancer are increasing in the U.S., due to the popularity of chewing and smokeless tobacco among younger men, says a report in *The Lancet* (2,8658:311).

Although lip cancer is detected easily (and treated more successfully than mouth cancer), most people wait too long before seeing a doctor. Long delays before treatment usually mean that the single, local cancer has spread to other areas. The big delay results in a five-year survival rate of only 30 percent.

Oral cancer is preventable: Stop smoking, decrease your alcohol intake and improve diet and oral hygiene. See your dentist regularly because oral cancer screening is part of a routine dental examination.

Now there's also news from a recent report from the National Cancer Institute that indicates if you eat more raw fruit you may lower your risk of getting cancers of the mouth and throat.

NCI researchers say that vitamin C, carotene and fiber present in generous amounts in raw fruits may be part of the reason for the protection, but not the only reason. They failed to find a similar preventive effect in vegetables, some of which also contain those same nutritional ingredients.

The study says that people eating more than four raw fruit servings every day have about half the oral cancer risk of people who average eating one or fewer servings daily. The researchers think the extra anti-cancer action may be due to the mechanical cleansing action of the raw fruit during chewing and swallowing. Another reason might be the presence in fruit of ellagic acid, thought to be a cancer inhibitor.

Just eating some cooked vegetables without fruit failed to lower the risk of oral cancers. But chewing crispy vegetables did have a beneficial effect, but not as much good effect as the multiple servings of raw fruit each day.

The same study says that drinking coffee and other hot beverages has no effect, either positive or negative, on mouth and throat cancer risks.

Vitamin A may prevent oral cancer

A recent study indicates that taking vitamin A or its "previtamin" form, beta carotene, may reduce the risk of getting oral cancer, even among heavy users of tobacco.

Scientists from the British Columbia Cancer Research Center in Vancouver gave weekly doses of 200,000 international units (IU) of vitamin A to 21 persons in a study in India. The persons studied all chewed tobacco mixtures and showed signs of developing oral cancers.

The treatment shrunk precancerous white spots (called leukoplakias) on the tongue and mucous lining of the mouth in 12 of the persons studied. The vitamin therapy also prevented new sores from forming during the year-long study. That degree of prevention over such a long period impressed the researchers, the report said.

The researchers worried about the possible toxic effects of megadoses of vitamin A over a year's time. Vitamin A is fat-soluble and is stored by the body. (On the other hand, vitamin C, which is water-soluble, passes quickly through the body and must be replenished daily.)

Continued overdoses of vitamin A can lead to serious health problems. To compare the vitamin doses involved, remember that the U.S. minimum dietary requirements of vitamin A for an adult add up to 35,000 IU in a week's time. The Indian patients received more than five times that amount every week.

The Vancouver scientists are looking for ways to avoid the overdose danger and still get the cancer prevention effects. One way, now being studied, may be to take smaller "maintenance" doses of vitamin A, the report said. Another may be to eat red palm oil, which is rich in beta carotene, the study said.

Using beta carotene to prevent oral cancer shows promising results in other research as well. A report on a study of beta carotene benefits was recently presented to the American Society of Clinical Oncology at a meeting in San

Francisco, says *Medical World News* (30,16:19).

In the study, each of 23 people with precancerous patches in their mouths received a 30-milligram daily dose of beta carotene. Within six months, the beta carotene treatment apparently caused the sore-like areas to shrink by half in 17 of the 23 people.

Beta carotene is a yellowish substance that the body converts into true vitamin A. You can reap beta carotene's anti-cancer benefits by eating more leafy, dark-green vegetables and deep-yellow fruits such as kale, spinach, carrots, peaches, papayas and cantaloupe, according to *Medical World News*. Normal servings of these sources can provide five to six milligrams of beta carotene daily. That allows your body to produce about one milligram of vitamin A, which is within the range recommended for good health, according to *The Merck Manual, 15th edition* (p. 900).

Previous studies have found that vitamin A-type compounds seem to fight formation of several kinds of cancers, including those of the larynx (voice box), esophagus, stomach and bladder. Ongoing studies are measuring beta carotene's potential for preventing lung and skin cancers.

Ovarian cancer

Milk sugar can be cancer risk for some

Women who have trouble digesting a form of sugar found in dairy products may face higher risks of developing cancer of the ovaries, a study in *The Lancet* (2,8654:66) suggests. The study is the first to link dairy products to ovarian cancer, says *Science News* (136,4:52).

The researchers "found that women who ate yogurt at least once a month were nearly twice as likely to develop ovarian cancer as women who reported less frequent yogurt consumption," according to the *SN* report. Eating cottage cheese at least once a month also raised the cancer risk, the report says. The culprit may be galactose, a type of dairy sugar, the researchers say.

Some women have trouble producing a digestive enzyme to break down the galactose, according to the study. Many don't even know they have the problem. But if they eat dairy products, this disability may result in "potentially toxic galactose bathing their ovaries for longer than women who metabolize the sugar efficiently," says the *SN* report. "Women who consumed more dairy products than they could metabolize had the greatest risk of ovarian cancer," the report says.

People get the bulk of galactose during digestion of lactose, the main sugar found in milk products. A little galactose is found naturally in most dairy products. But yogurt and cottage cheese contain higher amounts of galactose. That's because a natural bacteria process breaks down the lactose and releases galactose during the making of the two products.

If the surprising findings are backed up by other studies, "avoidance of lactose-rich foods by adults may be a way of primary prevention of ovarian cancer," says Harvard Medical School researcher Dr. Daniel W. Cramer, one of the authors of the study.

Pancreatic cancer

Amazing fish oil fights deadly cancer of the pancreas

New research suggests that a diet high in fish oil may do double duty in fighting cancer of the pancreas. First, the omega-3 fatty acid in the fish oil seems to prevent the formation of precancerous tumors, based on animal studies reported in *Science News* (135,25:390).

Second, the oil — from a common deep-sea fish called menhaden — also may hinder the spread of a tumor that's already turned into cancer.

Cancer of the pancreas is the fifth leading cancer killer in the United States. Scientists suspect that high-fat diets are a major risk factor for getting this disease. The pancreas is a banana-sized gland behind the stomach that produces digestive juices and hormones.

Researchers are finding out that the kinds of fats you eat could make a lot of difference in your cancer risk. For example, in one animal study, rats were injected with a powerful chemical that is known to trigger pancreatic cancer. The rats then were fed a high-fat diet containing either 20 percent corn oil or 20 percent fish oil, according to a report of the study published in the *Journal of the National Cancer Institute* (81,11:858).

The rats fed fish oil developed only about one-third as many precancerous tumors as the corn oil-fed rats, the report says. After tumors turned into cancer, the researchers were able to slow their growth and spread by lowering the total amount of fat in the diets.

"We are showing that using different (dietary fats), you can affect the progression of a cancer," says biochemist Reuven Reich in the *SN* report.

Other studies suggest that omega-3 (the short name for eicosapentanoic acid, found in abundance in cold water fish) itself slows down the spread of cancer cells from their original site to other parts of the body.

"There's no doubt about it. Something about fish oil puts it in a separate category from the average oil," agrees Leonard Cohen of the American Health Foundation in Valhalla, N.Y. But, he notes, you have to eat a "hefty" amount before seeing the anti-cancer effects.

How much omega-3 should be eaten daily is still up in the air. One recent nutrition study suggests that the government should develop a recommended minimum daily dietary amount for average Americans. No such RDA for omega-3 currently exists.

Many doctors recommend that you get the benefits of omega-3 oil by eating cold water fish rather than by taking capsule supplements containing fish oil.

People with diabetes and those who take aspirin or blood thinners or have recently had surgery should be especially careful about taking fish oil supplements.

The omega-3 acts like a blood thinner itself. Such combinations of blood thinners and fish oil could cause excessive bleeding.

Coffee and cigarettes:
A deadly combination

"Cancer of the pancreas is the fourth leading cause of cancer death in the U.S.," reports *The Western Journal of Medicine*.

Coffee has often been cited as a possible cause of pancreatic cancer. A recent study by five doctors in southern California did find a link between coffee intake and cancer of the pancreas, the *Journal* says. But the study showed that coffee drinkers who smoked faced the greatest risk.

Previous studies have focused on either cigarettes or coffee as risk factors. This controlled study, conducted in a county near San Diego, divided the coffee drinking participants into smokers and non-smokers.

Results showed that while the risk of pancreatic cancer is fairly low in those who drink less than four cups of coffee a day, those who both smoke cigarettes and drink coffee stand a much greater chance of getting pancreatic cancer.

Interestingly, the results were basically the same regardless of whether a person drank regular or decaffeinated coffee.

"This study is the first to show an effect of drinking

coffee on the risk of pancreatic cancer that is almost completely limited to cigarette smokers," the *Journal* concludes.

Skin cancer

Vitamin product prevents skin cancer

We know that the best way to prevent skin cancer is to avoid exposure to ultraviolet (UV) rays from the sun and in places like tanning booths. But some people at high risk may need to take further preventive action, doctors at Boston University School of Medicine report.

Five people with a rare skin disorder (xeroderma pigmentosum) that causes cancer took high doses of Accutane for two years. Researchers found that it completely prevented the development of skin cancer, according to *The New England Journal of Medicine* (318:25).

Accutane (generic name isotretinoin) is a strong, toxic derivative of vitamin A that is used to treat severe cases of disfiguring acne. It causes birth defects in pregnant women and is considered a drug of "last resort" in acne patients because of its serious side effects. The study said the researchers believe that if Accutane can prevent skin cancer, even in such a small study, some less poisonous form of vitamin A may be found that also can prevent the disease. The search is underway.

The good news for light-skinned persons or those with a family history of skin cancer is that the vitamin A-derivative approach is not just a treatment; it represents actual prevention of skin cancer among high-risk people.

Regular vitamin A is an absolutely essential part of a normal diet, necessary for eye health and good vision, especially at night. It helps the body resist respiratory diseases and shortens durations of several diseases. In normal amounts, it aids in keeping outer layers of tissues and organs healthy and promotes normal growth and strong bones.

Although the body stores vitamin A, men need about 1,000 micrograms to prevent deficiencies; women require about 800 micrograms daily. Some of the best natural sources include fish liver oil, liver, carrots (one cup of cooked, diced carrots contains about three times the RDA of vitamin A), green and yellow vegetables, yellow fruits, eggs, milk, and dairy products.

Don't take too much vitamin A. Daily megadoses of vitamin A of 20 times the RDA taken for several months can produce poisonous side effects.

Stomach and gastric cancer

Onions and garlic might be natural cancer fighters

You may not like what onions and garlic do to your breath. But your stomach and colon may be dying for what these members of the allium family can contribute to better health.

Scientists at the National Cancer Institute, working with colleagues in China, discovered that Chinese who eat a lot of onions and garlic have only a fourth as many stomach cancers as other Chinese. That's important, because the Chinese population has a high rate of stomach cancers, according to a report of the findings in *Healthline* (8,8:5).

Researchers are still trying to determine what it is about onions, garlic, chives, leeks and scallions that seems to slash the numbers of such deadly cancers. One NCI official suspects that the protective agent is the smelly part of the vegetables, the allyl sulfides, according to another report in *Health* (21,5:16).

Scientists at the University of California, Berkeley, think the answer may lie with a turncoat chemical, quercetin. Quercetin switches sides in the cancer battle, sometimes acting like a powerful cancer causer, other times like a strong cancer fighter. It's found in alliums and in deep green and yellow vegetables like broccoli and squash. It also turns up in red grapes and in common plants like ferns. Onions are extremely high in the substance.

In ferns and red wine (made from fermented grapes), quercetin seems to be a mutagen, a chemical that helps to trigger cancerous tumors. In fruits and vegetables, quercetin ties in with natural sugars and takes on a neutral stance, neither causing nor fighting cancer.

But once those sugar-linked quercetin molecules get into the digestive system, our natural enzymes break down the sugars and release quercetin into the stomach and intestines. Some bacterial enzymes present in our digestive tract act differently or not at all with different foods. For example, some bacteria work only with milk products. What quercetin does to our insides — whether it acts as friend or foe — may depend on what kinds of natural bacteria we have inside us and on what combinations of food we eat, the Berkeley scientists think.

Apparently, the alliums and quercetin act as allies against cancer. But researchers say more study is needed to see what exactly goes on. Meanwhile, consider adding more onions and garlic to your recipes, says the *Health* story.

Bitter is sweet cancer fighter

Don't make a face at that bitter taste when you eat citrus fruits. The natural chemical compounds that make the fruit slightly bitter also seem to have some cancer prevention qualities. That's the preliminary finding after researchers tested the compounds — called limonoids — on rats. They found the citrus bitters caused increased secretion of an anti-cancer enzyme in the rats' stomachs, giving them added protection against stomach tumors and stomach cancers. The report in *Nutrition and Cancer* (12,1:43) says the limonoids are found in oranges, lemons, limes and grapefruit, among others.

General cancer protection

Cabbages, collards and cancer

Several studies have shown that some common vegetables like cabbages and collards fight the formation of cancerous tumors. In particular, big cabbage eaters have higher than normal protection against cancers of the stomach, breast and colon. Animal studies showed increased protection against cancer of the lung for animals fed diets rich in cabbage and cauliflower.

Now, a study in the journal *Nutrition and Cancer* (12,2:121) demonstrates that a diet including cabbage and collards protects against the spread of breast cancer to the lungs. This study, involving rats, is the first to show that a diet that includes a particular family of vegetables fights the spread of cancer cells from its original location to another site in the body.

"The metastasis, or spread of a tumor to a secondary site, is the cause of death of a majority of patients, despite removal or treatment of the primary tumor with chemotherapy or radiation," the report says.

All the animals got injections of live breast cancer cells. Then the researchers watched to see how many in each group would develop cancer of the lungs as a result of the spread of the cancer cells. At the end of the two-month experiment, animals fed cabbages and collards had half as many lung tumors as the rats fed a control diet without the two vegetables. The researchers said they felt collards and cabbage diets might be useful in treating active cancerous tumors in addition to fighting the spread of the disease.

Cabbages and collards are both in a family known as cruciferous vegetables. Cruciferous vegetables get their name from the scientific term for plants whose flowers have petals in the shape of a cross. *Cruciferae* is the Latin name meaning "cross-bearing."

Among the many edible plants in this family are cabbage, cauliflower, collards, broccoli, brussels sprouts, kohlrabi, kale and radish.

B vitamins may offer protection from cancer

The B family of vitamins may fight tumor formation and boost protection from cancer, according to a nutrition scientist. That's important "because 30 to 40 percent of cancers in men and up to 60 percent of cancers in women are related in some way to diet," *Food and Nutrition News* (61,3:15) reports.

"The B-complex vitamins appear to have supportive roles in maintaining immune system functions which can aid in preventing growth of initiated tumors, as well as having anti-cancer effects of their own," researcher Ronald Ross Watson writes in *Food and Nutrition News*.

"A balanced diet consisting of moderate amounts of a wide variety of wholesome foods, including those containing the B-complex vitamins ... will enhance health and offer protection against the devastating disease of cancer," Watson says.

- Pyridoxine (vitamin B6) — "Of all the B-complex vitamins, vitamin B6 appears to have the most important role in maintaining the normal functioning of the immune system," says Watson. Deficiencies of vitamin B6 possibly decrease resistance to cancer and other diseases. In addition, vitamin B6 is being tested as a treatment for melanoma skin cancer.

- Folic acid — Increased intake of folic acid might decrease the occurrence of cancer, some researchers believe.

  That's because people with folic acid deficiencies have higher rates of stomach cancer and cancer of the esophagus, the tube from the mouth to the stomach.

  Folic acid supplements have also been used to successfully treat cervical dysplasia, a precancerous condition of the opening to the womb, according to *Food and Nutrition News*.

- Vitamin B12 — "A recent preliminary study in smokers who had potentially precancerous lung lesions implicated a role for folic acid and vitamin B12 in (lowering) the risk of lung cancer," Watson says. "Vitamin B12 is also thought to support immune system functions," he says, but its unique role is difficult to identify because vitamin B12 works and interacts so closely with folic acid.

- Thiamine (vitamin B1) — "Animal experiments have shown that a deficiency of thiamine may cause immune system impairment," and could play a possible role in the development of human cancer, the study reveals.

- Riboflavin (vitamin B2) — "Certain populations of people in China, Africa and Iran who have dietary deficiencies of vitamin B2 have shown a high incidence of esophageal cancer," according to Watson. Riboflavin is important in the development and maintenance of certain cells in the esophagus. In some cases, riboflavin supplements helped shrink cancer sores, but more research is needed in this area, he says.

  "Whole grains, nuts, beans, lean meats, milk, eggs and leafy, green vegetables are good sources of B vitamins," according to the article.

"The risk of cancer may be expected to be increased if people avoid certain healthful foods, such as dairy products, lean meats and nuts," just because these foods are high in calories or fat, Watson warns. In any diet you follow, make sure you get the recommended daily minimums of essential vitamins and minerals.

Natural cancer fighting strategies

Many health-conscious readers already know there's a lot of evidence showing that carotenoids (relatives of vitamin A), vitamin A itself, vitamin E, the mineral selenium, omega-3 in fish oil, and dietary fiber seem to protect some people from various kinds of cancers.

But there's more good news about some natural cancer fighters you may not have heard much about.

■ Getting more vitamin D may help people living in areas of high air pollution avoid cancers of the breast and colon, says a report in *Modern Medicine* (57,6:29).

Researcher Cedric Garland says excess sulfur dioxide in the air around industrial cities may block sunlight. Less sunshine means lower levels of vitamin D in the bloodstream.

Lower levels of serum vitamin D are linked with a five-fold increased risk of colon cancer and doubled risk of breast cancer, the report says.

After studying cancer rates in 35,000 men and women in Maryland and 18 Canadian cities, he recommends taking at least 400 IUs (International Units) of vitamin D each day.

That's the same as 10 micrograms (abbreviated either "mcg" or "μg") of cholecalciferol, the chemical name for vitamin D.

Instead of taking it in pill form, Garland's advice is to drink at least four glasses of vitamin D-enriched milk each day. That will give you the 400 IUs, he says.

Of course, as always, check with your doctor before taking any supplements or trying to medicate yourself.

■ Eating strawberries, grapes and Brazil nuts may help your body ward off cell damage from cancer-causing chemicals known as carcinogens, according to researchers at the Medical College of Ohio in Toledo.

Many kinds of nuts and berries contain ellagic acid, says scientist Gary D. Stoner in *Science News* (133:216).

Ellagic acid snoops out cancer-causing chemicals floating in the bloodstream and neutralizes them, the report says.

In tests on mouse and human lung tissue, the nutty substance also seems to help keep normal cells from becoming cancerous, Stoner reports.

But it only works when added to the system just before or during the time the body is exposed to the carcinogens, the report says.

Supplements of pure ellagic acid don't work well, Stoner says, because the body has trouble absorbing the concentrated version.

The natural stuff, in nuts and berries, is the most easily absorbed form, he says.

■ Cheese, milk and even some kinds of cooked meats — including charbroiled hamburgers — contain a substance that burrows into your body tissue and sets up anticancer guardposts inside the cells themselves, according to researchers at the University of Wisconsin-Madison.

The anticancer substance is a form of linoleic acid, a kind of fatty acid present in large concentrations in cheese and grilled ground beef, says a report in *Science News* (135,6:87).

Linoleic acid is one of three polyunsaturated fatty acids that seem to be very efficient killers of cancer cells, the report says.

But since this form of linoleic acid comes buried in a food's fat — including the saturated kind that can load up your blood with high levels of cholesterol — researchers advise against pigging out on cheese and hamburgers just to get the anticancer effect.

"But within a balanced diet... [linoleic acid] may confer some protection against cancer — particularly when present in combination with other dietary anticancer agents... found in many vegetables, including beans, rice and potatoes," the report concludes.

■ You kitchen veterans will recognize this common spice, easily found at your neighborhood grocery store.

It's the yellow stuff — known as curcumin — found in the spice turmeric, that seems to halt tumor growth, to prevent new tumors from forming and to hunt down and neutralize cancer-causing chemicals in the blood, says a report in *The Journal of the American College of Nutrition* (8,5:450).

Turmeric is peppery and sometimes is substituted for saffron.

It's used in curry recipes, on rice dishes, with yellow vegetables and, in Europe, even as coloring in some beverages like lemonade.

■ More spicy anti-cancer agents include ginger and clove, reports the Oct. 25, 1990 issue of *The Atlanta Journal.*

Animal studies show that these spices might help fight cancerous tumors.

But, don't go overboard with the spices. Small amounts are all that is necessary. For example, you don't even need a quarter of an ounce of ginger each day to get the health benefits it provides.

■ Besides being good sources of nutrients, raw broccoli, cabbage, cauliflower and brussels sprouts also contain cancer-preventing compounds.

But notice that they should be raw, not cooked, say

researchers at the University of Manitoba in Winnipeg.

That's because cooking, especially in water, drains the cancer-fighters out of the vegetables, says the report in *Science News* (136,22:351).

These leafy vegetables — members of the Brassica family — contain lots of anti-cancer compounds called indole glycosinolates.

The compounds prevent breast tumors and precancerous sores inside the stomach in animal tests, the report says.

Indole glycosinolates also tr_gger release of enzymes that take the sting out of cancer-causing chemicals in some foods we eat, according to the report.

■ By the way, don't use soap to wash your vegetables before eating, warn government health officials.

Soap leaves unseen residues on your vegetables, which can cause intestinal problems, says Myron Johnsrud of the U.S. Department of Agriculture.

Best way to clean your vegetables: rinse thoroughly under plain running water, says USDA.

■ Several animal studies suggest that diallyl sulfide and other sulfide compounds in garlic fight growth of cancerous tumors in the colon, lung and esophagus (the 9-inch food tube from the mouth to the stomach).

Of course, garlic is well-known as a folk remedy for all sorts of ailments. But there have been very few tests to determine whether its anticancer qualities in animals hold true in people, the report says.

That may change soon. The National Cancer Institute is studying 10 garlic compounds to see if they are safe for human tests.

If they are, and if they prove out in scientific trials, the next step could be "garlic-fortified" cereals, the report predicts.

General cancer risks

Too much iron may cause cancer

Iron supplements should be avoided unless people have a deficiency, new research suggests. A recent report says unusually high doses of iron have been linked to greater human cancer risks.

A report in *The New England Journal of Medicine* (319:1047-52) warns that excess amounts of iron stored in the body may cause an increased risk of cancer and death, particularly in men. In a study involving 14,000 people over 13 years, the researchers linked high body levels of iron with cancer of the colon, bladder, esophagus and lungs.

Unlike most other vitamins and minerals, iron is not automatically thrown off by the body, but is stored. Therefore, taking too much iron can cause unhealthy iron deposits in the body.

People with low levels of iron in their blood, known as anemia, often take several iron supplements daily. Supplements also are recommended after surgery, blood loss, for people with hemorrhoids, peptic ulcers, or colitis, or for women with heavy menstrual periods. The U.S. government also recommends extra iron for women during pregnancy and breast-feeding. Additional iron is very important for the health of these people.

However, other people take iron as part of their daily vitamin and mineral intake, or just because they feel that more iron will help keep them healthy. But iron supplements for people who are not anemic may be unwise, Richard G. Stevens, Ph.D., stated in the journal.

Many foods, like breakfast cereals, often have added iron. Because of the possible link with cancer, Stevens questioned whether everyday foods should be "iron fortified."

Common U.S. fern linked to high cancer rates

The bracken fern, one of the world's most common plants, has been linked to cancer in animals who eat it and to high rates of cancer in people who live or work in bracken-covered areas, the *Medical Tribune* (30,6:2) reports.

Two field guides to edible wild plants in America recommend eating this plant, either cooked or raw. A recent report from Europe, however, accuses the same plant of being a potent cancer-causer. "Deer, cattle and sheep that graze on bracken develop mouth and stomach cancers," the article says.

Studies from Costa Rica and Venezuela showed that people who drink milk from cows that have grazed on bracken, in turn, develop more cancers of the stomach and esophagus, the *Tribune* article says.

The fern under fire is known scientifically as *Pteridi-*

um aquilinum and is commonly known in this country as pasture brake, eagle fern, brakes, hog brake and brake fern. It is the single most common wild fern in the United States.

It grows easily in "full sunlight, in woods, old pastures, new roadsides, burned-over regions, sandy and partially shaded areas and in thickets," according to *Field Guide to Edible Wild Plants* (Stackpole Books, 1974: page 158), a manual still being sold in many bookstores.

Still another manual, *Field Guide to North American Edible Wild Plants* (Outdoor Life Books, 1982: page 58) lists bracken as a "related edible species" to ostrich fern. In that guide, bracken was considered a non-poisonous plant.

Even getting close to bracken might be hazardous, the *Tribune* report suggests. One expert recommends that anyone who goes often into areas in which bracken covers the ground should wear a face mask to limit exposure to bracken spores.

The spores are thought to contain several powerful cancer-causing substances such as shikimik milk, quercetin and ptaquiloside.

That face mask group should include "shepherds, forestry workers, and even hikers and backpackers," according to Dr. Jim Taylor of University College in Wales (Great Britain) and chairperson of the International Bracken Group.

"People may also be affected by drinking water from bracken-covered slopes" and by drinking milk from cows who have eaten bracken, he warns.

Bracken is one of the first ferns to appear in the spring.

It grows to a height of from one to four feet, adding new leaves throughout the warm months. The darkly green fronds look heavy and leathery.

The fern spreads by oozing a toxic chemical into the ground that poisons all surrounding plants competing for the same space. These same poisons can affect both animals and people, according to the *Tribune* report.

The potentially dangerous spores are released from the maturing plant from June through October, Taylor says.

A further note — much research has been done on cancer-causing chemicals in recent years. Anyone who relies on field guides for safely stalking wild asparagus and other such wild delicacies should be sure the material has been printed very recently and contains the most up-to-date scientific information.

Check with your doctor or an expert in plant-produced chemicals about questionable plants. Safest bet of all—if it's wild, don't eat it. And, in the case of bracken fern, don't even get near it.

Warning: This drink might cause cancer

A potent carcinogen called urethane is present in hundreds of alcoholic beverages, the *Nutrition Action Health Letter* says. Worse, no one seems to know how to remove it from the beverages.

According to government tests, the most highly contaminated are bourbon whiskey and fruit brandies. "But many dessert wines, table wines and liqueurs are also tainted," the *Letter* adds. The Food and Drug Administration has yet to publicize the names of brands containing urethane.

The Center for Science in the Public Interest (CSPI), however, has put out a booklet entitled "Tainted Booze," which lists the levels of contamination in over 1,100 brand name products. It also answers questions about urethane. The booklet's author, Charles Mitchell, says that although the whiskey and wine industries have agreed to lower levels of urethane in their future products, they are still too high.

"There is no evidence that any safe level of urethane can be ingested without increasing the risk of cancer," he adds.

So far the whiskey and wine industries' agreement to set limits on the amounts of urethane they put in their products is voluntary; there is no way of assuring they stick to their guns. Also, the agreements do not protect consumers from urethane-contaminated booze now being sold, the *Nutrition Action Health Letter* points out.

CHAPTER 15

Colitis

Dietary help for colitis sufferers

The term colitis refers to a number of diseases, all characterized by inflammation of the colon—the lower and biggest part of the large intestine. The inflammation can cause gas, stomach cramps, frequent trips to the bathroom and bloody stools. In severe cases, a person may be unable to pass waste from the body.

According to the *Tufts University Diet and Nutrition Letter*, the exact causes of colitis are not known. Treatments therefore sometimes differ. Many doctors, however, agree that dietary treatments can be extremely helpful.

The *Tufts University Letter* recommends a low-fiber diet for colitis sufferers. Raw fruits and vegetables, bran and whole grains should be cut back sharply if not entirely. Such measures will lessen irritation of the colon. (It is hoped they will decrease the frequency of bathroom visits as well.) Nutritional supplements might also be needed, the *Letter* adds. When suffering from colitis, a person might have little appetite and therefore might not be consuming adequate nutrients through food.

The *Saturday Evening Post* recommends a dairy product-free diet for colitis sufferers. Many colitis victims suffer from a reaction to lactose in dairy products, which they don't digest properly.

CHAPTER 16

Depression

A vitamin deficiency might lead to depression

Low levels of the B vitamin, folic acid, have been linked to depression by A. Missagh Ghadirian of McGill University in Montreal (as reported in *Psychosomatics*).

Dr. Ghadirian found that folic acid supplements relieved depression in people whose depression was caused by low folic-acid levels. Depression, loss of appetite, dizziness, fatigue, and shortness of breath are the first signs of a folic acid deficiency.

Folic acid is a water-soluble vitamin, so extra amounts are usually passed out through the kidneys into the urine within 24 hours. Without regular folic acid, deficiency symptoms may occur after just 100 days of low folic-acid intake. Adults require 400 micrograms of folic acid daily. In addition, pregnant women need 800 micrograms to help prevent birth defects. Nursing mothers should have 500 micrograms each day.

Folic acid is found naturally in yeast, liver, lima beans,

whole-grain products, leafy, green vegetables, oranges, asparagus, turnips, peanuts, oats, potatoes and beans. Folic acid dissolves in cooking water when foods are heated, so raw foods are a better source of this vitamin.

Many things can interfere with the body's proper absorption of folic acid. Even if you are getting the daily requirement, your body might not be able to use it. Oral contraceptives, aspirin, acetaminophen (like Tylenol and Panadol), Dilantin, primidone, phenobarbital, methotrexate, pyrimethamine, triamterene, and high doses of vitamin C reduce the amount of folic acid available for the body to use.

The percentage of depressed people who are actually suffering from a folic-acid deficiency is not known, the report said.

CHAPTER 17

Diabetes

Maturity onset of diabetes and obesity

Elevated blood sugar levels create major problems for individuals with diabetes.

Dietary fiber seems to step in and stop this problem. Fiber appears to slow the release of sugar into the bloodstream. Without this huge influx of sugar, the body doesn't suddenly need to produce insulin.

This may help prevent diabetes from developing in individuals who would otherwise develop the disorder. It might also reduce the amount of medication needed by insulin-dependent individuals.

Insulin, as you will recall, is a type of hormone. It takes the sugar molecules in the blood and guides them to the cells where they may be burned up as fuel.

In a Kentucky study, a doctor placed people with adult-onset diabetes on a diet rich in carbohydrates and high-fiber foods. As the diet took effect, the diabetics needed 25 to 100 percent less insulin than they were using prior to their new, high-fiber diet.

These dietary changes also help people who are over-weight.

Individuals on high-fiber diets are rarely fat. For practical reasons, the extra fiber helps make you feel full, without adding lots of calories. Also, many high-fiber foods, especially vegetables, take longer to chew.

The effects of fiber on insulin are also factors for people who are obese.

Because a person on a high-fiber diet is less likely to have sudden peaks of blood sugar and insulin, she is less likely to feel hungry as quickly after a meal.

Without the fiber, hunger pangs begin sooner, resulting in more food consumption. Eating more than is needed results in obesity.

Poor dietary habits may add up as you get older, and your hormone levels, including insulin, naturally drop off. When that happens, obesity and unnatural eating habits put too much of a load on your pancreas, and you might become susceptible to developing diabetes.

A proper diet now might reduce your chances of coming down with diabetes later in life.

However, if you already have diabetes, be sure to check with your doctor before you change your diet.

The doctor may have you on insulin, and any change could upset the carefully balanced carbohydrate requirements that he may have specifically developed for you.

Also, some cases of diabetes are not caused by diet or obesity. In juvenile diabetes there is a lack of insulin, possibly caused by a viral attack on cells that produce it.

A better sweetener?

Diabetics and dieters, have you ever wanted a sweetener that is safe, sweet and tasty? Well, thanks to Danish scientists, you may soon have one, says *The American Journal of Clinical Nutrition* (52,4:675).

The Jerusalem artichoke can provide a kind of natural sugar called fructan that might fulfill all of your requirements for a sweetener.

This new sweetener has two main benefits:

1. Low in calories. Fructan has long molecules instead of the short molecules found in most common sugars. Your body cannot absorb the long fructan molecules very well. This means that you may take in a lot of calories by using the sweetener, but you won't have to suffer the consequences because your body can't "use" the sugar.

2. Stabilizes blood sugar levels. Fructan does not appear to cause a drastic change in blood sugar levels.

Eating carbohydrates usually raises blood glucose levels.

But, when fructan is used, the blood sugar levels appear to be lowered instead of raised.

And fructan seems to reduce the body's need for insulin, which is great news for diabetics.

Scientists are still researching and studying fructan, but some forms of fructan are already on the market.

If you are on a special diet or are taking insulin or other

medicines, check with your doctor before using fructan products.

High-carbohydrate diet might be risky for diabetics

To lower heart-disease risk, the American Heart Association (AHA) recommends a low-fat, high-carbohydrate diet for all Americans. Some researchers contend a high-carbohydrate diet might be harmful for people who are insulin-resistant — namely, diabetics — who cannot process large amounts of carbohydrates (*Science News*, 136,12:185).

Both the AHA and the American Diabetes Association (ADA) recommend that carbohydrates make up 50 to 60 percent of daily caloric intake. Some researchers believe that percentage is too high.

"When patients who have non-insulin-dependent diabetes are given this so-called 'good' diet, they have marked increases in triglycerides [a form of fat in the bloodstream] and a significant decrease in HDL cholesterol [high-density lipoprotein, or "good" cholesterol]," says diet researcher Ann M. Coulston of Stanford University. "And in patients with diabetes, a rise in triglycerides is associated with an increased risk of cardiovascular disease."

Coulston advocates a diet of 40 to 45 percent total carbohydrates. She and her colleagues conducted a six-week study, giving 12 diabetics two diets for six weeks at a time. Carbohydrates made up 40 percent of total calories in the first diet, and 60 percent in the second (the recommended amount).

"Diabetics on the 60 percent diet had a 30 percent rise in serum triglycerides and a 9 percent decrease in HDL," according to Coulston's report at the ADA meeting last June.

The ADA hasn't been quick to change its dietary guidelines, however. It will wait for further research to confirm these results.

A little table sugar might be safe for some diabetics

There may be good news on the horizon for some diabetics. Adding sucrose to their restricted diets had no bad effects on a small group of Type-II (non-insulin-dependent) diabetics, according to an Australian study. Sucrose is a natural sweetener that most of us know in its refined form as table sugar.

"Our study suggests that the controlled use of sucrose can be considered in certain [diabetic] individuals," researchers report in *The American Journal of Clinical Nutrition* (50,3:474). The results of this and other studies may redefine the traditional dietary guidelines for diabetics.

Diabetics cannot process natural sugars efficiently. So, until now, they have been told to avoid table sugar completely. Diabetics regularly use artificial sweeteners such as aspartame, which is why researchers chose it for study.

They studied nine people whose diabetes was well

under control. None were taking insulin, and all were in good health. Three were treated with diet only, and six were treated with diet and a drug used to control diabetes.

Researchers randomly assigned participants to one of two groups for six weeks each. One group received one and one-half ounces of sucrose daily, and the second received about five and one-half ounces of aspartame, the amount equivalent in sweetness to sucrose. The participants did not suffer any harmful effects from the supplements and were able to process sugar effectively, even without the drug.

Total cholesterol, high-density lipoprotein (HDL or "good") cholesterol and triglycerides (a type of fat in the bloodstream) "were not significantly different" at the end of each study period, compared with the levels measured before the study began. The same held true for blood-sugar and insulin levels.

Researchers "caution against overinterpreting the results," emphasizing the following:

- The form of sucrose used is important. Participants used sucrose as an additive, only in coffee or tea or on breakfast cereal. High-fat, high-sugar baked goods were not evaluated.
- Participants must be followed up for long-term side effects.
- Regular "diabetic-type" diet is important. Studies in which sucrose supplemented a high-carbohydrate diet had poor results.
- The study size was small, only nine people. Much larger studies are necessary for more precision in

determining accurate results that might apply to most Type-II diabetics.

If you are a diabetic, don't try this experiment on your own. Check with your doctor before making any change in your diet or treatment program.

Pass the pasta to conserve chromium and avoid diabetes

The spaghetti you eat today may help keep you healthy tomorrow! Researchers now believe that eating a diet that conserves the mineral chromium may prevent the development of a form of diabetes called Type-II diabetes.

This form of diabetes usually affects adults over forty who are overweight. The people who risk developing this non-insulin-dependent form of diabetes are not able to absorb the blood sugar (glucose) from their bloodstreams properly and are said to be "glucose-intolerant."

Your doctor can give you a simple test that will reveal whether you have mild glucose intolerance, the condition that precedes Type-II diabetes. If you are mildly glucose-intolerant, don't worry! You may still be able to avoid diabetes with certain changes in your diet.

The key is to increase the amount of chromium in your body. According to *Science News* (137,14:214), chromium can improve your ability to use blood sugar and help prevent the development of Type-II diabetes.

Unfortunately, it's not that easy to increase your chromium. You can eat high-chromium foods like meat, cheese, whole-grain breads and cereals, broccoli, potatoes, and some fruits, wines and beers. But your body can't easily absorb the chromium from all these natural sources.

Researchers suggest another approach to try in combination with a chromium-rich diet: stay away from foods rich in simple sugars such as fructose and glucose. These foods cause your body to excrete large amounts of chromium.

On the other hand, eating foods that are high in complex carbohydrates, such as pasta, will help you conserve the chromium in your body.

Ask your doctor's advice. If you have mild glucose intolerance, or even if you have already developed Type-II diabetes, you may be able to improve your glucose tolerance just by changing your diet.

Magnesium helps lower blood pressure in Type-II diabetes

You've heard the old saying that "an apple a day keeps the doctor away."

The next verse could go something like this: "A fresh salad a day helps keep hypertension away."

It seems that eating a fresh, green salad with lunch every day might help lower your blood pressure if you suffer from high blood pressure and Type-II diabetes.

What's so great about a green salad? you ask.

Green, leafy vegetables found in fresh salads are good sources of the mineral magnesium. Magnesium is an important mineral in the human body, and studies show that a magnesium deficiency may contribute to high blood pressure, reports *Science News* (138,12:189).

Eating green vegetables every day helps increase the amount of magnesium in the body. And a magnesium-enriched diet might help lower high blood pressure by relaxing constricted (tightened) blood vessels.

Recent studies suggest that people with high blood pressure and Type-II diabetes have low levels of magnesium in their red blood cells.

So, researchers think that many Type-II diabetics could help control their high blood pressure by taking magnesium supplements or by eating foods rich in magnesium.

However, they warn that magnesium supplements could be dangerous for some diabetics.

Apparently, some people with diabetes can experience kidney problems that could result in dangerously high levels of magnesium in the blood. Therefore, researchers recommend that all diabetic people consult their doctors before taking any magnesium supplements.

Peas for diabetes

Meet the newest fiber on the health food block — pea fiber.

Yep, pea as in English peas, or field peas.

Danish researchers say the kind of dietary fiber found naturally in peas helps smooth out the usual sharp rise in blood sugar levels right after a meal.

That's good news for diabetics, especially, because they sometimes have trouble controlling what's called postprandial (after-meal) glycemia (high levels of blood sugar).

An added bonus: used in regular baked products, the pea fiber tastes okay, too, says the report in *The American Journal of Clinical Nutrition* (50,2:324).

The researchers compared the beneficial effects of a commercial brand of pea fiber available in Denmark to comparable amounts of wheat bran and beet fiber.

"The postprandial blood-glucose response was markedly reduced by the (pea fiber)," the report says. "Because the palatability is good, it may prove a valuable food additive for diabetics."

The wheat bran and beet fiber had almost no effect on either blood-glucose or serum-insulin levels, the researchers say.

The pea fiber used is a white, almost tasteless, granulated powder that is easily baked into bread, the report says. About two-thirds of pea fiber is the water-soluble type.

The added pea fiber had no effect on normal bowel movement schedules, the study says.

Only one patient reported any side effects: a feeling of fullness after eating the test meal containing 30 grams (just over one ounce) of pea fiber in a mixture of ground beef and two kinds of sugar.

Low protein for diabetics

A low-protein diet can reduce the chances of further kidney damage for diabetics and other people with kidney diseases, researchers report in *The Lancet* (2,8677:1411).

For years, doctors have advised diabetics to eat the same amount of protein as healthy people.

But now they're saying that too much protein could stimulate more blood flow into the kidneys, making them work harder. This extra strain on the kidneys could be dangerous.

You have a better chance of avoiding kidney damage if you follow a low-protein diet in the early stages of a kidney disease, researchers say.

Low-protein diets cannot stop kidney damage in the late or final stages of a serious kidney disease, they add.

In a British study of 19 people in various stages of kidney disease, a low-protein diet reduced stress on the kidneys and slowed kidney damage.

Similarly, an 18-month Australian study of 64 diabetics showed that restricting protein intake delays kidney damage.

Half of the group ate their regular diet, while the other half ate a protein-restricted diet.

Nine of 33 people on the regular diet developed kidney failure, compared with only two of 31 people on the protein-restricted diet.

Although a low-protein diet seems to be the best way to protect kidneys from further damage, be very careful about changing your diet.

A drastic change may do more harm than good.

Your doctor or nutritionist can help you plan a safe and healthy diet to suit your nutritional needs and give you the best possible results.

CHAPTER 18

Digestive Health

Diverticular disease

Diverticular disease is a painful inflammation of pouch es in the walls of the large intestine.

The pouches may develop because of the force the colon has to exert to push along the large, hard masses of waste that result from a highly-refined diet.

This pressure causes abnormally high force on the walls of the colon. Eventually, little ballooning pockets form in the intestinal wall, in which fecal matter can lodge and cause infection.

Diverticulosis is the name of the condition that happens when the intestine develops pouches. Diverticulitis is the name given to an infection or inflammation of one or more of these pocket-like areas.

Many doctors who treat people with diverticular disease now recommend that they eat a diet high in dietary fiber or that they take a fiber supplement. The types of fiber recommended are the mushy types such as psyllium seed products or oat bran, as well as whole-grain products. Hard types of fiber such as popcorn should be avoided.

Symptoms of diverticular disease usually clear up when people follow a doctor-prescribed, high-fiber diet. However, the weakness that caused the pockets in the wall of the colon will remain.

Individuals with diverticular disease must truly change their diet for life.

Symptoms of the disease may return if patients don't follow a high-bulk diet faithfully or don't take a psyllium mucilloid fiber supplement. Although the problems caused by diverticular disease will not disappear, in most cases, they can be minimized and controlled so that surgery or antibiotic treatment can be avoided.

Rice bran reduces colon cancer risk

Researchers at the Royal Hallamshire Hospital in Sheffield, England, recently compared rice bran and wheat bran.

"The results of this study indicate that rice bran is an efficient stool bulking agent," said J. Tomlin, leader of the research team, as reported in *European Journal of Clinical Nutrition* (42:857-61).

Even though volunteers only ate a slightly larger amount of rice bran, "it increased stool mass and frequency by over twice the increase caused by wheat bran."

The more bulk created in the stool and the faster the

waste can be moved from the intestines, the lower the incidence of colon cancer. Rice bran is a type of dietary fiber that decreases the risk of colon cancer because it helps move waste products through the intestines rapidly.

With less contact with the lining of the intestines, the cancer-causing contents in the intestines seem to be less harmful.

In a separate study in Japan (*Journal of Nutritional Science Vitaminology*, 32:581-89), researchers compared a brown rice diet to a diet of polished rice, where the bran was removed. "The results suggest that rice fiber produced an increase in fecal weight, which is assumed to be effective in preventing colonic disease in advanced countries," the researchers concluded.

Your fiber intake should be at least 30 grams each day and include a variety of fiber types, according to the National Cancer Institute. "Dietitians recommend a high-fiber diet for patients with cardiovascular problems, obesity and diabetes, diverticulitis, and gastrointestinal problems or diseases," according to Babcock. For more on prevention, see the colon cancer section.

How to put brakes on breaking wind

Benjamin Franklin called it, "Breaking wind." Some say, "Passing gas." The technical term is flatulence, and it has been the source of everything from off-color fraternity jokes to serious attacks of pain—and social embarrassment — for some sufferers.

Almost everybody experiences up to a dozen episodes daily of passing gas. It's the normal by-product of healthy digestion. Unfortunately, in some cases, that gas also can become trapped in folds of the colon and cause mild to severe pain.

"It may feel like a knife stabbing the chest or abdomen," says Dr. John H. Renner. Because the pain can be severe and occurs in areas close to the heart and stomach, many sufferers fear the pain may signal more serious problems like heart disease and ulcers, even cancer.

The gas itself is caused by fermentation, the same process that makes wine. Bacteria are normally present in the digestive tract, according to a report from the American Digestive Disease Society. When the bacteria work on the undigested parts of a big meal, one by-product is a mixture of gases, including hydrogen sulfide (the familiar rotten-egg odor) and smelly residues of fatty acids.

Several things contribute to excess flatulence and gas pain, Renner says. Here are the main ones:

(1) The kinds of food we eat. Almost everybody gets gas from eating beans. That's because beans contain two kinds of starches that bacteria love to ferment and that the body can't break down and absorb first. Other problem foods include onions, brussels sprouts, raisins, prune juice, apricots, celery, carrots, bananas, bagels, wheat germ and pretzels, not necessarily in that order.

Sometimes a combination of otherwise innocent foods will trigger excess gas. Keep track of what you eat, compare that with when you experience gas discomfort, and tailor your diet accordingly.

For example, one would not want to eat a large plate of beans or brussels sprouts just before attending a play that contained extended quiet periods. On the other hand, such precautions might not apply before a rock concert.

(2) Sudden switch to more high-fiber foods. Most of us need more fiber in our daily diet. But one of the prices we have to pay may be increased flatulence.

"Start with a small dose of fiber so the bowel gets used to it," advises Dr. Michael Mogadam of Georgetown University. "That lessens the increase in flatus." After about two weeks on an increased fiber diet, most people's gas production returns to normal levels.

(3) Lactase deficiency. Some people lose the ability to digest milk and milk products efficiently because of a shortage of a digestive enzyme, lactase. Undigested milk sugar gets to the colon and becomes a ripe target for gas-producing bacteria. Try a milk-free diet for two weeks to see if episodes of excess gas decrease. Your doctor can help you zero in on the cause.

Old-fashioned candy relieves gas

An old-time favorite candy, peppermint, may relieve stomach gas. Thomas L. Kun, a California gastroenterologist disclosed in *Prevention* magazine that peppermint helps to release intestinal gas.

Peppermint allows the sphincter muscle at the base of

the esophagus to relax, and as this happens stomach gas is released. If someone swallows a lot of air when he eats and he feels bloated, relaxing this muscle will relieve his indigestion.

Taking eight drops of spirit of peppermint (available from your pharmacist) in warm water, drinking peppermint tea made from real peppermint leaves, or eating mints made with genuine oil of peppermint are good sources of peppermint recommended by this gastric specialist.

One word of caution is given about this remedy: If you have a tendency toward heartburn, you should avoid this treatment. It may mean your sphincter muscle is so weak that it is allowing acid out of your stomach. In this case, the sphincter muscle should remain as tense as possible, so you should avoid peppermint.

Bananas for indigestion pain?

Bothered by indigestion pain? Eat a banana!

That's the essence of a study by researchers in India, reports *The Lancet* (335,8689:612).

They took 40 people — each of whom had experienced many months of stomach pain and nausea but who had no ulcers — and tried a natural remedy on half of them.

The researchers gave 20 of them capsules containing banana powder—eight capsules a day for eight weeks. The second group of 20 took nothing for the discomfort. All of them stayed away from antacids or ulcer medicines.

By study's end, half of those who took banana pills

reported complete relief, and another one-fourth received at least some relief from their constant indigestion problems.

In the other group, eight out of 10 still had indigestion problems.

Bananas are a common food in India, and many Indians also use banana powder, a dried and ground-up form of the fruit, the report says.

Banana powder also protects the stomach lining from irritation by aspirin and some other drugs, say the report authors, and has been used with some success in treating ulcer symptoms. No side effects were reported.

Try iced tea instead

Hot drinks, such as tea and coffee, can give you an ulcer, British researchers report in *Gut* (30:1201, 1989).

The hotter the drink, the more damage done to the protective lining of the stomach.

The lining protects the stomach from acid attack.

Spice for life

Ginger is believed by some to be one of the better natural stomach "medicines" around.

Ginger seems to help prevent stomach ulcers, says a digest in *HerbalGram* (20:23).

It also is used commonly to prevent or calm motion

sickness, morning sickness, or just general nausea.

How to avoid 'stomach flu'

What you assume to be stomach flu is probably food poisoning, says Patricia Long, salmonella expert. Long says technically that there is no such thing as stomach flu. Usually, the guilty organisms have entered your body through water or mishandled food.

The salmonella bacteria "are the number-one cause of food-borne illness in the U.S.," Long says. She warns that "no turkey is fully cooked" and that too often chickens and turkeys are removed from the oven too soon and left to sit at room temperature. This encourages bacteria to flourish and multiply like crazy.

Long notes that over one-quarter of the chickens consumed by Americans are contaminated with the salmonella bacteria. Although 40,000 cases of salmonella food poisoning are reported each year, Long estimates as many as 4 million go unreported. "Most of these illnesses begin in our own kitchens," she says.

Common advice on how to avoid salmonella includes not allowing frozen foods to thaw by leaving them outside the refrigerator or not leaving prepared foods out for over two hours.

Based on studies Long has conducted with the Infectious Disease Program of the University of California's School of Public Health, she discovered that undercooked fowl, particularly the stuffing in turkey, are covered with bacteria that multiply quickly when left outside the oven for long.

"Given the chance, salmonella will live in almost anything edible," Long says, "but they prefer high-protein foods like meat and eggs. Foods with a lot of salt, sugar or acid, such as dry salami, jams, jellies, soy or citrus marinades and yogurt, will slow down the bacteria from multiplying."

For example, Long says that contrary to popular belief, store-bought mayonnaise will not cause poisoning because it "has enough salt and acid to inhibit bacterial growth." Chocolate candy and milk, on the other hand, contain little salt or acid and will actually protect the bacteria from stomach acid.

Symptoms of salmonella infection will occur within 12 to 48 hours and include nausea, diarrhea, abdominal cramps, fever and headache. Vomiting will occur on occasion.

Once you've got it, the best advice is to "drink fluids, stick to a bland diet and wait it out," Long says. Most have no idea it was salmonellae that hit them, unless the infection is severe enough to require a hospital visit. In such cases, "antibiotics may be prescribed to prevent bacterial invasion of the brain (meningitis), the lung (pneumonia) or the joints (arthritis)," Long reports. While these complications are rare, the Center for Disease Control in Atlanta estimates there are 500 to 1,000 deaths each year due to salmonella poisoning.

Long concludes the best prevention is to "assume that all meats are tainted, then prepare, cook and store foods with care," she says. Also, keep work spaces and sponges clean and watch out for microwave ovens. They often cook unevenly and bacteria may exist on uncooked portions of food.

Microwaving might contribute to food poisoning

British researchers believe they may have found a hidden danger in microwaving prepared foods. The amount of salt or sugar in these foods may change the way the foods absorb microwave energy, says a report in *Science News* (137,14:215).

Researchers found that a high salt or sugar content prevents foods from reaching a high enough temperature to kill salmonella and other dangerous bacteria. In fact, microwaving may only heat these bacteria to a temperature that helps them grow rather than kills them.

To avoid food poisoning, researchers agree that you should microwave foods longer and at a lower temperature than the package recommends. Then let the food sit for a few minutes to make sure dangerous bacteria have been killed.

Relief from diarrhea

The most important thing you can do if you're suffering from diarrhea is to replace the fluids your body is losing, says a report in *Medical Abstracts* (10,2:2). Even if you're nauseated and sick at your stomach, you need to try to force some liquids down.

Try to take frequent small sips of liquids such as Gatorade; fruit drinks; chicken broth without fat; and non-diet, non-caffeinated soft drinks.

Try to drink at least two quarts of liquids a day. And drink three quarts if you have a fever, the report suggests.

CHAPTER 19

Dizziness

A diet for dizziness

Dizziness can be caused by your diet, according to Dr. Joel Lehrer at the New Jersey University of Medicine and Dentistry. About 90 percent of people who suffer from dizziness can be helped by a simple change in diet.

Some people's bodies don't properly absorb food, and this can cause dizziness, Dr. Lehrer explains.

In a study, he tested a change in diet to 50 percent of calories from complex carbohydrates, like rice and spaghetti, 30 percent from fats, and just 20 percent from protein. He found that such a change seemed to reduce or eliminate dizziness in people he studied.

The amount of food and calories consumed should be based your age, height, weight and body frame, but it's the breakdown of calories that is important.

Changing to large amounts of complex carbohydrates, small amounts of lean meat and using only polyunsaturated fats might make a big difference in your life.

However, most diabetics and hypoglycemics will not

be helped by this diet because their dizziness is not caused by this mechanism.

CHAPTER 20

Ears and Hearing Problems

If you once prided yourself on your keen sense of hearing, but you now find yourself asking people to repeat things, you might need some more vitamin A in your diet.

Some cases of hearing loss might be linked to a vitamin A deficiency, *The Journal of Nutrition* (120,7:726) reports.

Studies show that a lack of vitamin A in the diet first increases the ear's sensitivity to sound. In other words, with this vitamin deficiency, your hearing is actually better at first.

However, an increased sensitivity to noise increases the chances of noise-induced hearing loss. The very-sensitive ear can be damaged more easily and quickly than a normal ear.

So, the vitamin A deficiency does not actually cause the hearing loss. It simply makes the ear more sensitive to sound—which increases the chances of hearing loss due to noise damage.

If you suspect you may have a problem with your hearing, talk to your doctor immediately. He can help you determine whether you need more vitamin A in your diet.

CHAPTER 21

Fatigue

A mineral you might be missing

If you are getting adequate sleep each night but still feel "draggy," your body might be trying to tell you something. You might have an iron deficiency.

Unusual whiteness of the palms of the hands or the eyelids might be an early sign of iron deficiency. Lack of iron causes tiredness and is especially common in women. However, the *British Medical Journal* reports that tiredness sometimes is a symptom of advanced iron deficiency. If people with unusually pale palms or eyelids take iron supplements, a serious iron deficiency can be avoided. Women with heavy menstrual periods or those who are using intrauterine devices (IUDs) require more iron. Anyone who is suffering from fatigue might benefit from taking extra iron.

Whole-grain products, liver and organ meats, red meat, eggs, lima beans, prunes, spinach, raw broccoli, peas, fish and raisins are all good natural sources of iron. Iron supplements should be taken with food, orange juice or meals.

Avoid taking iron supplements with tea, coffee or milk, since these beverages reduce absorption of iron into the body.

Feeling weak? You might need more of this nutrient

Have you ever been so weak you had trouble just getting up in the morning? A woman recently felt that way, and neither she nor her doctor could determine the reason.

Not until the woman was tested for deficiency of a certain mineral did the cause become apparent: her body was starved for potassium, a nutrient plentiful in bananas and oranges.

Millions of Americans are deficient in potassium. Among those at high risk are people like this woman who take diuretics for high blood pressure. While extracting salt and fluid from the body, diuretics can also remove potassium.

Lack of potassium manifests itself in tiredness and sluggishness, and causes leg cramps and irregular heart-beats.

The woman's doctor brought her potassium level back to normal with potassium supplements. Eating enough bananas and oranges should now maintain that level.

Pep without pills

Fatigue may be a symptom of a serious disease that

needs medical treatment. A physician should be consulted if fatigue continues.

Fatigue might be caused by a deficiency of certain vitamins or minerals, including thiamine (vitamin B1), riboflavin (vitamin B2), niacin (vitamin B3), pantothenic acid (vitamin B5), vitamin B12, vitamin C or folic acid.

Over-consumption of caffeine may cause fatigue when the effects of the drug wear off, especially early in the morning. Monitor the number of caffeine-containing drinks (colas, coffee, tea) that you have daily, and start eliminating them.

Taking vitamin E in doses larger than the recommended daily dietary allowance (RDA) is reported to sometimes cause fatigue.

Taking extra vitamin C or the mineral manganese has been reported to reduce fatigue in some people.

CHAPTER 22

Fish Oil and 'Fishy' Plants

Grandma was at least partly right when she dosed you with cod liver oil for whatever ailed you.

You and grandma may not have realized it, but after the bad taste left, an all-natural ingredient in the oil went to work in your bloodstream.

It began working to lower cholesterol levels in your blood, improve the health of your arteries, and reduce your risk of heart attacks and strokes caused by blood clots.

Most doctors don't recommend cod liver oil for their patients anymore because it also contains cholesterol. But, an increasing number of researchers and physicians are discovering the many healing benefits of that natural ingredient, now called omega-3 fatty acids by scientists and simply "fish oil" by the rest of us.

The insides of arteries suffer injuries, sometimes from turbulent blood flow. Sticky platelets in the blood collect around the injured area and send chemical signals for more sticky helpers, including germ-fighting white cells. The result, sometimes, is too much help.

Cholesterol, a natural part of blood, collects in unusual amounts at the growing bottleneck in the busy blood pipeline. The "helpers" continue to send signals that cause more of the blood's clotting agents to pile on the growing mass. The result is atherosclerosis: a form of hardening of the arteries caused by fatty plaque growing on and changing the walls inside arteries.

These plaque blockages reduce blood flow, especially in arteries feeding the heart. Reduced blood flow, in turn, starves whole areas of heart muscle, resulting in heart pain (angina) or even heart attacks. Plaque blockages also cause blood clots to form, further reducing blood flow. That can happen in many areas of the body besides the heart.

And healing apparently is what omega-3 does inside blood vessels. Omega-3 fish oil helps the healing process by making the blood helpers less sticky, and by keeping them from piling up and blocking the artery.

It helps in a second way, too. One part of the fish oil, EPA (eicosapentaenoic acid), gets into the cells that make up the artery walls. The EPA-fortified cells start cranking out their own chemical signals that order sticky, clot-forming platelets to stay away.

"Increasing fish oil in the diet leads to a slight lowering of cholesterol (of the harmful LDL type), and it sometimes reduces high blood pressure as well," reports Dr. Alexander Leaf, writing in *Your Good Health*, a publication of Harvard Medical School.

But that's not all. Other studies suggest fish oil helps the joints, cuts down on arthritis discomfort, and reduces the pain of and even prevents migraine headaches (*Total Nutrition Guide*, Bantam Books, pg. 43).

More recent animal studies (*Science News*, 134:228) indicate that well-fed mice on high-fat diets that included fish oils rich in omega-3 —

(1) Lived twice as long as normal mice.
(2) Had half the normal levels of harmful autoimmune responses (inflammatory diseases like rheumatoid arthritis and lupus, in which antibodies attack the body's own tissues).
(3) Showed a complete absence of kidney disease, which normally strikes all these kinds of test animals.
(4) Had blood cholesterol levels half that in normal mice, even lower than those in another study group of mice that had been fed calorie-restricted, low-fat diets.

Researchers are now testing fish oil in people to see what effect it has under clinical conditions on several other diseases. These problems being researched include psoriasis, nephritis (inflammation of the kidneys), lupus, arthritis, and some forms of cancers involving the immune system.

Eating fish is better

Although you can get fish-oil supplements (usually

sold as omega-3 in capsule form), many physicians say a safer way is to forget the pills and eat fish containing the oils. Eating fish avoids two common, unpleasant side effects of taking fish oil capsules — a bad aftertaste and burping.

The highest levels of the two kinds of beneficial fish oil ingredients (EPA and DHA fatty acids) are found in fresh or frozen fish that normally live in deep, cold waters. Eating canned fish is not recommended, since the canning process destroys most of the omega-3 oil.

Best of the saltwater breeds are mackerel (Atlantic, king and chub), Pacific and Atlantic herring, European anchovies, chinook salmon, sablefish, sturgeon, tuna and mullet.

Cod is a cold-water fish, but has relatively little omega-3 oil in its flesh. Instead, the cod stores omega-3 in its liver. But many doctors advise against a regular supplement of cod liver oil, since too much of the old remedy can cause overdoses of vitamins A, D and E.

Among freshwater fish, highest omega-3 levels are found in lake trout and whitefish. Shellfish like lobster, crab and shrimp have smaller amounts of omega-3, as do mollusks like scallops and clams.

Fish oil's Top 20

Based on an uncooked serving size of 100 grams (approximately three and one-half ounces), the following kinds of fish are highest in total omega-3 fatty acids content.

Fish	Total fat in grams	Total omega-3 fatty acids in grams
Atlantic mackerel	13.9	2.6*
Chub mackerel	11.5	2.2
King mackerel	13.0	2.2
Lake trout	9.7	2.0
Japanese horse mackerel	7.8	1.9
Pacific herring	13.9	1.8
Atlantic herring	9.0	1.7
Bluefin tuna	6.6	1.6
Albacore tuna	4.9	1.5
Sablefish	15.3	1.5
Chinook salmon	10.4	1.5
Atlantic sturgeon	6.0	1.5
Lake whitefish	6.0	1.5
European anchovy	4.8	1.4
Atlantic salmon	5.4	1.4
Round herring	4.4	1.3
Sockeye salmon	8.6	1.3
Sprat	5.8	1.3
Bluefish	6.5	1.2
Mullet	4.4	1.1

*About one-tenth of one ounce

Source — U.S. Department of Agriculture, Human Nutrition Information Service

Veggies have it too

Don't like fish that much? You can still get some omega-3 through plant sources, according to *Everyday Health Tips* (Rodale Press, pg. 74). But, most plants generally are lower in omega-3 than the same amounts of fish. However, there are exceptions.

For example, oat germ is a good source of omega-3, better than all but 15 kinds of oil-rich fish. Three and one-half ounces of oat germ has more omega-3 than the same amount of sockeye salmon or mullet.

Common dry beans have more omega-3 than ocean perch, Pacific halibut, red snapper and many other kinds of fish. The lettuce-like purslane, used in soups and salads in Mediterranean countries, is high in EPA. Also good are tofu, walnuts, wheat germ oil, several kinds of beans, soybean products and rapeseed oil.

Margarine also is a rich source of omega-3, largely because it's made from soybeans. Unfortunately, it also has more saturated fats than fish or other plant sources of omega-3.

Best plant sources of omega-3

The following are plant sources high in omega-3 fatty acids. The comparisons are based on a serving size of approximately three and one-half ounces (100 grams).

Food	Total fat (in grams)	Omega-3 (in grams)	Omega-3 as % of fat
Rapeseed oil	100.0	11.1	11.1
Walnut oil	100.0	10.4	10.4
Wheat germ oil	100.0	6.9	6.9
Soybean oil	100.0	6.8	6.8
English walnuts	61.9	6.8	10.9
Black walnuts	56.6	3.3	5.8
Tomato seed oil	100.0	2.3	2.3
Soybeans, sprouted, cooked	4.5	2.1	46.6
Dry soybeans	21.3	1.6	7.5
Oat germ	30.7	1.4	4.5
Leeks, raw	2.1	0.7	33.7
Radish seeds, sprouted	2.5	0.7	28.0
Wheat germ	10.9	0.7	6.4
Common dry beans	1.5	0.6	40.0
Navy beans	0.8	0.3	37.5
Pinto beans	0.9	0.3	33.3
Kale, raw	0.7	0.2	28.5
Spinach, raw	0.4	0.1	25.0
Strawberries, raw	0.4	0.1	25.0

SOURCE: U.S. Department of Agriculture, Human Nutrition Information Service

RDA for fish oil?

Here's an imaginary question — have you had your minimum daily requirement of fish oil today?

It's imaginary because right now there's no such thing as a Recommended Dietary Allowance (RDA) for omega-3 fatty acids.

In what may be the first such official argument, Norwegian researchers are suggesting that a minimum level should be established for "essential fatty acid," just as there are standards currently for vitamins, minerals and other basic nutrients. (In Europe, what we call our RDA is known as the MDR (Minimum Daily Requirement).

Their suggestion is reported in *The American Journal of Clinical Nutrition* (49:290-300).

The Norwegian researchers, led by Kristian Bjerve, discovered that omega-3 fatty acids are essential for the normal metabolic processing of another kind of dietary oil, omega-6 fatty acids.

Omega-6 oils are close relatives of omega-3 oils and are found in things like safflower oil and other cooking oils.

The Norwegians found a direct relationship between daily doses of omega-3 oils and healthy levels of certain blood substances.

In their study, they found that 350 to 400 milligrams of omega-3 acids in the form of purified fish oil are needed daily to maintain normal plasma and lipid levels.

"Omega-3 fatty acids possibly also have some specific function in the retina (in the eye) and in the central nervous system," Bjerve says.

"Dietary fish oils are rich in eicosapentaenoic acid (EPA), a polyunsaturated fatty acid of the omega-3 series," according to *Postgraduate Medicine* (85,4: 406).

Essential fatty acids, like EPA, have been discovered to play important roles "in the control and prevention" of heart and artery disease, the lowering of high blood pressure and preventing unnecessary blood clotting.

Current research is also investigating fish oil's potential to help in angina (heart pain), rheumatoid arthritis and other inflammatory disorders, kidney disease and breast cancer, *Postgraduate Medicine* reports.

Another study at the Pennington Biomedical Research Center in Baton Rouge, La., found that fish oil's anti-clotting action in animals "depends on the dosage of fish oil in relation to other kinds of polyunsaturated fats — not the absolute amount of fish oil consumed," *Science News* (135,12:183) reports.

"If confirmed in humans, the finding may lead to recommendations on how much of the different kinds of polyunsaturated fats people should consume," says the *Science News* report.

Since a daily requirement has not been set, and safe levels of fish-oil supplements have not been established, "the consumption of fresh fish two to three times weekly is likely a reasonable recommendation," says the *Postgraduate Medicine* report.

However, "deep-fried, smoked, overcooked, pickled, and salted fish should be avoided."

Remember that canning also destroys some of the omega-3 acid content, so fresh or frozen fish — the kind caught in deep, cold waters — are better sources of EPA than canned fish.

Best dose?

About three grams a day, or a little under one ounce a week, of omega-3 fatty acids — commonly known as "fish oil" — is the best dose size for cutting levels of fat in the blood, say researchers in *The American Journal of Clinical Nutrition* (52,1:120).

In a Dutch study, researchers at Amsterdam's Free University Hospital tested the effects of four different dosages of omega-3 oils on several types of cholesterol and triglycerides, as well as on the germ-killing power of white blood cells.

The doses tested ranged from zero to six grams a day. It takes 28 grams to make one ounce.

Triglycerides are a form of fat carried by the blood. Scientists consider high levels of triglycerides to be a risk factor for heart disease.

They found that fish oil even in small doses reduces triglycerides and raises the concentration of HDL ("good") cholesterol.

The effect was dose-dependent, meaning that the more fish oil taken by the volunteers, the more the benefits.

Up to a point, that is. Above three grams of fish oil per day, the body seems to be unable to use the extra fatty acids in a beneficial way.

Feeding the volunteers six grams per day had no more

effect than giving them three grams a day, the researchers report.

Some cautions

Some people shouldn't take fish-oil supplements or eat higher than normal amounts of food containing EPA and DHA.

Those with diabetes, persons with a history of hemorrhaging or strokes, or patients facing surgery or on aspirin and blood-thinning therapy should avoid fish oil unless specifically authorized by their doctors.

Fish oil can decrease the blood's ability to form clots. In addition, some people report heartburn and belching as sideeffects of taking fish-oil capsules.

Check with your doctor before taking any omega-3 supplements.

A natural way to get the benefits of omega-3 is to eat cold-water fish two or three times a week, suggest many nutritionists.

CHAPTER 23

Gallstones

Fish oil not only helps reduce heart-disease risk by lowering cholesterol, but it might also help prevent gallstones, according to researchers at the Johns Hopkins University School of Medicine and reported in *Science News* (135:21;332).

Gallstones — actually, cholesterol "crystals" — form in the gallbladder, a pouch located near the liver. A substance known as bile flows from the liver through the bile duct to the gallbladder, where it is stored and used for digestion. If gallstones lodge in the bile duct, surgery is sometimes needed.

A main "ingredient" of bile is liquid cholesterol.

Researchers don't know how liquid cholesterol hardens into gallstones, but they believe that omega-3 fatty acids found in fish oil halt the process.

Researchers recently tested their theory on prairie dogs. They fed 16 animals high-cholesterol diets; half were given fish-oil supplements.

After two weeks, researchers removed the animals' gallbladders.

The eight animals given fish oil had no gallstones; the other eight did.

Researchers are hopeful humans will show the same results. They plan more studies.

Chapter 24

Headache Helps

Little-known causes of migraine headaches that you can easily avoid

Do you suffer from occasional or chronic migraine headaches?

There's a good chance they can be avoided by eliminating particular foods from your diet, according to *Prevention* magazine.

A recent study, according to *Prevention* magazine, found allergies were responsible for migraine headaches in twenty-three of thirty-three sufferers. Each patient was allergic to an average of three foods. "Elimination of the guilty foods," *Prevention* reports, "brought headache relief, often within two weeks."

The offending foods included milk, cheese, eggs, chocolate, tea, tomatoes, coffee, shellfish, oranges, fish, wheat, rice and apples. Tyramine, the allergen in chocolate and "highly fermented cheese" is the most common culprit.

The researchers think headaches are probably triggered by "food substances causing sensitization of brain cells, which react to releasing histamine."

Natural ways to manage your migraine

People with migraine headaches should avoid food containing tyramine. Tyramine dilates the blood vessels and contributes to causing many headaches. Avoid certain foods in the following groups because they contain high concentrations of tyramine:

- meat and fish — chicken livers, sausages, pickled herring, dried fish and beef
- dairy — aged cheese, sour cream and yogurt
- alcohol — red wine, champagne, sherry, beer, ale, Riesling and sauterne wines
- vegetables — sauerkraut and fava beans (broad Italian beans)
- flavorings—chocolate, soy sauce, vanilla, yeast and nitrites

Nitrates are also known to cause certain types of headaches. Watch for nitrate or nitrate additives on product package labeling. Be sure to avoid:

- hot dogs
- bacon
- sausage
- pepperoni
- salami
- ham
- all processed luncheon meats
- all cured meat

Many people have severe headaches after eating food containing monosodium glutamate (MSG). MSG is often used in Chinese cooking, and these headaches and associated symptoms have been referred to as the Chinese Restaurant Syndrome. If you suffer from headaches after eating Chinese food, stop eating at Chinese restaurants or discuss with the chef the availability of MSG-free foods. MSG is also found in some meat tenderizers and many convenience foods—canned and frozen. Be sure to read the labels.

A promising new natural treatment for migraines is to take magnesium supplements. Magnesium is usually deficient in the American diet, and magnesium supplements like magnesium chloride or dolomite, which is composed of calcium carbonate and magnesium carbonate, are quite helpful to many migraine sufferers, especially women who suffer from migraines during pregnancy or near the end of their monthly cycles.

Dietary sweetener causes headaches

Studies have shown that diet "is an important element in the migraine headache process," according to the journal *Headache*. Chocolate, milk products, sherry and red wine have all been found to trigger migraine headaches, the journal says.

Evidence now suggests the popular dietary sweetener aspartame is the latest offender.

In a recent study at the University of Florida, aspartame

was discovered to increase frequency of headaches, the journal reports.

A group of people suffering from periodic migraine headaches took a 300-milligram capsule of aspartame four times a day for four weeks. Another group ingested a placebo (a neutral pill containing no chemical). After a one-week "wash-out" period the subjects switched; the aspartame group now took the placebo. During the eight weeks, the subjects kept a record of their food intake and frequency of headaches, designating types (migraine, tension, etc.) and how disabling they were.

The study concluded that "ingestion of aspartame by migraine sufferers might cause a significant increase in the frequency of migraines," according to the journal *Headache*. In addition, headaches were found to last a little longer when the subjects were taking aspartame, and several subjects had increased symptoms of dizziness, shaky feelings and poor vision during headaches. Aspartame was not found to increase the intensity of migraines, however.

The researchers note that with aspartame fast becoming the dietetic sweetener of choice in America, there are fewer and fewer products a migraine headache sufferer can safely use.

Caffeine: Friend or foe in headache relief?

Caffeine might provide relief from some people's headaches, but it can cause headaches in other people! How can this be?

According to Harold Gelb, D.M.D., in the book *Killing Pain Without Prescription*, drinking one or two cups of coffee may help constrict the blood vessels and reduce some people's headaches. However, constricting the blood vessels can cause headaches in other people, and withdrawing from habitual use of caffeine often causes headaches for a few days. Before you try coffee, tea, or other caffeine-containing products for headache relief, be sure you know if you are sensitive to caffeine.

Re-leaf for headache pain

Using herbal "medicines" to relieve common aches and pains is not just old folklore. Some scientists say that herbs may be just as helpful and useful in treating illnesses as modern medicine.

One such herb, called feverfew, may help cut the number and severity of migraine headaches you've been experiencing.

A digest report in *Science News* (134:106) suggests that taking daily capsules of ground feverfew leaves reduces migraine headache discomfort and also helps relieve the nausea that sometimes accompanies migraine headaches.

However, you should check with your doctor before trying any herbal supplement.

CHAPTER 25

Heart Health

Can you reverse coronary heart disease by eating your veggies, walking more, quitting smoking, relaxing and making new friends?

Yes, suggests an article in *Geriatrics* (45,12:73).

The one-year experiment divided 41 men and women, all of whom had suffered coronary heart disease, into an experimental group and a control group.

The experimental group underwent radical lifestyle changes, while the patients in the control group were given the conventional advice regarding lifestyle changes.

In other words, the control patients were told they could make changes in their lifestyle if they so desired.

The patients in the experimental group reduced their angina (chest pain) frequency by 91 percent; their angina duration, 42 percent; and their angina severity, 28 percent.

Those in the control group made modest lifestyle changes, but their angina frequency, duration and severity all increased.

The study also indicated that the sickest patients made the greatest improvements, and those improvements seemed to occur more readily in women.

The lifestyle changes included:

- Eating a vegetarian diet, which derived only 10 percent of its calories from fat.
- Managing stress by means of stretching exercises, breathing methods, meditation and progressive relaxation, at least one hour each day.
- Giving up the use of tobacco products.
- Exercising—usually walking—to 50-80 percent of individual target heart rates at least three hours a week.
- Gathering twice a week for group discussions to provide social support.

Natural ways to fight coronary heart disease

Many researchers recommend the following natural methods for treating or reducing the chances of developing coronary heart disease (or coronary artery disease):

- Reduce the amount of fat in your diet—especially reduce saturated fats, which are usually found in meat and dairy products. The American Heart Association recommends that saturated fats comprise only 30 percent of total calorie intake;

others suggest even lower levels of only 10 to 15 percent. These levels are substantially lower than the levels found in typical American diets. In a simplified form, this means eating less meat, dairy products, eggs and other sources of saturated fats and cholesterol, while relying more on starches and low-fat sources of protein, such as broiled fish and poultry.

Diets high in protein, as from meat, and low in lysine, as from low-fat dairy products, can contribute to heart disease.

- Eat saltwater fish more often. The omega-3 oil found in some freshwater fish and many saltwater fish has been shown to be beneficial in raising HDL levels in the blood. Recent population studies show that people who eat substantial amounts of cold water fish like trout, salmon, mackerel or cod have lower rates of coronary heart disease than other people, even if the total amount of fat in the diet remains about the same. These new studies suggest that the addition of fish to the diet, and especially the replacement of much red meat and dairy products with fish, could reduce the chance of developing coronary heart disease.

Snack for your heart

Snacking during the day, sometimes called "grazing," may be better for your heart than eating three square meals a day, Canadian researchers report in *The New England Journal of Medicine* (321,14:929).

But that doesn't mean you can eat just potato chips and ice cream — or simply snack between meals.

To get the benefits, you must eat small, nutritious meals throughout the day, researchers say, and your calorie count must not increase.

Researchers believe snacking works by controlling the production of certain chemicals in the body.

Insulin, a hormone released by the pancreas, helps the body produce cholesterol. How much insulin the pancreas releases into the bloodstream depends on the size of the meals you eat.

Snackers may have lower cholesterol levels because they eat smaller amounts of food, and the pancreas produces less insulin in response.

Less insulin usually means less cholesterol.

Eating more meals throughout the day and adding more fiber to your diet might be keys to keeping your cholesterol levels under control.

During the study, seven men aged 31 to 51 ate three meals a day for two weeks or 17 snacks a day for two weeks and then switched to the other diet.

The snackers' insulin levels dropped by 28 percent during the study.

Their total cholesterol levels were 8.5 percent lower

than men eating three meals a day.

Based on the results of this study, researchers believe that nutritious nibbling throughout the day may help you lower cholesterol levels and fight heart disease.

Vitamins and minerals that help your heart

In addition to the well-known therapies for preventing heart problems, here are some facts you should know about how specific vitamins and minerals affect your heart.

A pyridoxine (vitamin B6) deficiency may contribute to coronary heart disease. Pyridoxine supplementation may be especially helpful in preventing heart and artery disease for people who eat high-protein diets. When meat is cooked, it loses much of its pyridoxine, which could have been used by the body to help break down by-products of methionine, one of the amino acids found in protein. By-products of methionine are thought to damage the arteries and cause heart disease much like the process which is involved to a much greater extent in homocystinuria (an hereditary enzyme-deficiency disease). Taking supplements of small amounts of pyridoxine with each meal containing cooked meat may help to prevent some coronary heart disease.

A magnesium or selenium deficiency might result in coronary heart disease. People living in areas where these minerals are deficient in the water supply have high rates of heart disease.

When niacin (vitamin B3) is taken in high dosages, it has

been shown to reduce the amount of cholesterol in the blood (*Journal of the American Medical Association*). In a study of heart attack victims, it was found that people who took high doses of niacin had an 11 percent lower death rate than those who did not.

Niacin must be administered in high doses to be effective against heart disease and cholesterol. But, because of the significant side effects of large doses of niacin, it should be taken only under a doctor's supervision. Some people, such as those with high blood pressure, diabetes, gout or ulcers, should not take niacin at all. The niacinamide form of the vitamin should not be used because it does not lower blood fats by a significant amount. Food sources for niacin include yeast, fish, poultry, liver, meat, whole-grain products (except corn which contains an inactive form of niacin), peanuts, potatoes, beans and mushrooms.

People receiving digitalis or other heart medication should not take calcium ascorbate (a vitamin C formulation) since irregular heartbeats may occur.

Studies by Kurt A. Oster, M.D., and others indicate that folic acid might be helpful in the treatment and prevention of heart disease. Larger, controlled studies are necessary to confirm these studies.

Another medical doctor states that folic acid might stop the progress of coronary heart disease by neutralizing xanthine oxidase, an enzyme found in milk fat that may be harmful to the arteries, and by restoring a substance which repairs damage to arteries and helps stop the fatty buildup which is found in hardening of the arteries.

Beta carotene helps cut heart problems in half

Yellow might be the color of a healthy heart.

Yellow, that is, in the form of beta carotene, also known as previtamin A, the nutrient that gives the yellow color to carrots and squash.

Taking a 50-milligram dose of beta carotene every other day for six years seemed to help slow artery clogging in male doctors who already had heart disease, according to *Science News* (138,20:308).

Compared to men who took placebo (fake) pills, the beta carotene group had half as many "major cardiovascular events," such as heart attack or stroke, during the long-term study, according to another report of the Harvard Medical School findings in the *Medical Tribune* (31,24:2).

Researchers took into account that the beta carotene men also were taking aspirin on alternate days. The 333 randomly selected participants were drawn from the much larger Physicians' Health Study. This is the study that already has produced the discovery that an aspirin every other day protects against heart attacks.

Doctors still can't say whether otherwise healthy people would reap a heart benefit from taking beta carotene.

About 11,000 men in the large study have been taking the previtamin-A supplements. Final results will be available later this decade.

Scientists guess that beta carotene hinders the formation of a harmful kind of low-density lipoprotein (LDL) cholesterol. LDL cholesterol is known as "bad" cholesterol because of the damage it sometimes does to arteries.

Once linked with oxygen in the bloodstream, the harmful kind of LDL cholesterol probably damages artery walls, leading to plaque buildup.

Like sticky putty in a pipe, the plaque deposits choke off blood flow in arteries, resulting in heart attacks and strokes.

Beta carotene, they speculate, apparently derails that process in some way.

The beta form of carotene is just one of nearly 500 carotenoid compounds occurring naturally in vegetables and fruits. The various carotenes are responsible for the yellows, oranges and reds in carrots, mangoes, papayas and apricots.

Besides those foods, other natural sources of beta carotene include broccoli, winter squash, asparagus, spinach, sweet potatoes and cantaloupe.

Beta carotene is known as previtamin A because the body converts it into active vitamin A. Vitamin A, like other fat-soluble vitamins, is stored in the body. It's easy to overdose on vitamin A.

On the other hand, it's hard to get too much beta carotene, since the body converts to vitamin form only what it needs, disposing of any excess beta carotene.

The only bad side effect of even large doses of beta carotene is a yellow-tinged skin. But even that disappears when the beta carotene intake is reduced to normal levels.

The Recommended Dietary Allowance (RDA) for vitamin A for men over 50 is 1,000 micrograms, or one milligram, daily. For women over 50, it's 800 micrograms.

A lot of your daily vitamin A comes in the "preformed"

version in foods, ready to be used and stored by the body immediately, without conversion.

If you got your RDA of vitamin A strictly from beta carotene, you would need to take in from four to six milligrams of beta carotene daily.

For example, a half cup of cooked carrots contains nearly 12 milligrams of carotene, mostly the beta type.

The 50 milligrams of beta carotene taken daily by the members of the study group is about four times the amount normally found in a half cup of carrots.

The daily study supplement was well within the "safe" range, the *SN* report noted.

However, it's best to check with your doctor before taking supplements of beta carotene or any other nutrient.

Fish oil and heart surgery

Recent studies suggest that fish oil taken before and after two very different kinds of surgery can have highly beneficial effects. In one study, fish oil seemed to help keep arteries unclogged after "balloon" surgery. In another, fish oil apparently helped prevent the spread of cancer cells that escaped after operations.

An extremely high intake of fish oil can "dramatically improve" the results of coronary angioplasty, popularly known as "balloon" surgery, according to one new study at the Washington Hospital Center. Usually about one-third of arteries opened with angioplasty get clogged up again with cholesterol and plaque within six months. But Dr.

Mark R. Milner said his research suggests that taking large doses of fish oil for just six months can cut that failure rate in half.

Fish oil seemed to help patients after another kind of surgery, as well. A Harvard Medical School study suggested that highly purified fish-oil supplements helped prevent spread of cancer cells that may escape during and after surgical operations to remove cancerous tissue.

Dr. George Blackburn of Harvard, who's also chief of nutrition support at New England Deaconess Hospital, said the fish-oil supplements were given to cancer patients a week before surgery. Following surgery, the patients continued taking the fish oil for three to six months. Blackburn noted lower rates of cancer spread, known as metastasis, in those who took fish oil.

Both doctors have a very conservative approach to fish-oil therapy for all but these two classes of surgery patients. Milner advised against taking fish-oil capsules for any other reason, because, he said, the long-term effects are still unknown. "I never give fish-oil supplements to any of my patients unless they are having coronary angioplasty," he said. Blackburn recommended eating deep-water fish four or five times a week, rather than taking fish-oil capsules.

In the fish-oil study on heart patients, 194 persons were randomly assigned to two groups following successful angioplasty. One group took nine fish-oil capsules per day for six months after the procedure. Each capsule contained a total of 4.5 grams of omega-3 fatty acids. That's about the daily equivalent of the fish oil in two cans of sardines.

The other group got no fish oil, but patients in both

groups were told to eat low-fat, low-cholesterol diets. Both groups received the same post-operative therapy. Nurses trained in diet therapy called each patient monthly to provide counseling and to evaluate if the patients were sticking to their strict diet.

"Dietary compliance was equally good in both groups of patients," Milner noted. "They really tried to stick with a strict low-cholesterol diet." Patients' cholesterol intake was restricted to 100 milligrams per day, and dietary fat was limited to 25 percent of their total calories.

By the end of six months, 35.4 percent of people who didn't take the fish oil showed signs that their dilated heart arteries had narrowed again. However, the recurrence rate in the fish-oil group was only about 19 percent, Milner reported.

During the study, eleven patients stopped taking the high doses of fish oil because of disagreeable, but not dangerous, side effects, including flatulence and other mild digestive problems. Milner said that most patients were willing to tolerate the side effects in order to possibly lower their risk of having a repeat angioplasty or needing bypass surgery.

Coronary angioplasty is less invasive than heart bypass surgery because it does not involve cutting open the chest cavity. Instead, the surgeon cuts into a leg or arm artery and inserts a catheter with a tiny balloon on the tip. He threads the narrow catheter through the circulatory system until its tip reaches the portion of the heart artery that is narrowed by fatty "plaque." Then the doctor inflates the balloon, squashing the plaque against the artery wall and enlarging the inner diameter of the blood vessel. Several blockages can be opened during the procedure.

Since the use of angioplasty began more than a decade ago, scientists have been searching for a drug to reduce the procedure's failure rate.

Aspirin has proven to be helpful in reducing the number of heart attacks that happened during or soon after angioplasty. But aspirin doesn't seem to make a significant difference in reducing the six-month reclogging rate, known as "restenosis," said Milner, who is assistant professor of medicine at George Washington University.

Milner's findings are similar to the results of a smaller study of 82 patients at the Dallas VA Medical Center, reported in *The New England Journal of Medicine*. Milner said several research teams are doing comparable studies to confirm these results.

Fish oil seems to suppress the inflammatory response that follows an injury, Milner said. In angioplasty, the inner wall of the artery is sometimes injured by the balloon catheter. If the injured area heals rapidly, excess inflammation, scar tissue and blood clots may combine to clog the artery again. Fish oil seems to slow the unwanted speedy healing process and to prevent the inflammation and scarring. It also seems to reduce the tendency of blood platelets to form clots at the once-clogged site.

The outer membranes of almost all cells contain oils called omega-6 fatty acids. "Overdosing" patients with fish oil high in omega-3 fatty acids alters their cell membranes. Omega-6 fatty acids in the membranes are replaced by omega-3 fatty acids. This change seems to make cell membranes less "reactive," Milner said. Thus, a person whose cell membrane content is high in omega-3 fatty acids may have white blood cells that are slower to cause inflammation and red blood cells that are slower to form clots, both good effects for heart health.

After your first heart attack...

Eating fish at least twice a week might prolong your life, according to a new study in *The Lancet* (2,8666:757).

Even people with advanced heart disease could benefit, the two-year study suggests.

During a two-year study, 2,000 men who had suffered their first heart attacks received advice about fat, fish and fiber intake.

Those men who ate fatty fish — such as mackerel, herring, salmon and trout — or took fish-oil supplements reduced their chances of dying from another heart attack by nearly one-third.

Those in the less-fat group had no added benefits, while those who ate more fiber actually showed a slight increase in fatal attacks.

Although eating fish didn't cut the number of new heart attacks, it seemed to cut the number of fatal attacks, the study indicates.

Researchers believe fish oil helps prevent clogged arteries, though it may take as long as two years to see any positive effects.

They plan more long-term studies.

Coffee and caffeine: How much is too much?

If you're worried about your cholesterol levels or suffer from cardiovascular disease, put down your cup of coffee and take note. Research indicates that drinking one to five cups of caffeinated coffee every day nearly doubles your risk of heart disease and strokes, compared with non-coffee drinkers, according to *U.S. Pharmacist* (14,6:28). Six cups a day of the regular brew increases your risk 2.5 times, the report says.

A "safe" daily intake of caffeine is about 200 milligrams (less than one-hundredth of one ounce), according to the report. But one regular cup of coffee contains at least 170 milligrams.

Excess caffeine can provoke arrhythmia, an irregular heartbeat. That can be dangerous for some people. Too much caffeine also seems to be linked to increased levels of blood cholesterol, which in turn can be very bad for your heart and arteries.

In one eight-week study, patients with existing heart rhythm problems got worse after taking the equivalent of three to five cups of caffeinated coffee each day, says a report in *American Family Physician* (39,6:214).

Researchers haven't managed to tag coffee with directly causing cancer. But, they point out, heavy users of caffeine also tend to be heavy smokers. Tobacco smoking has been established to be a proven, direct cause of lung cancer. As for other cancers, "It appears that coffee drinkers are marginally more likely to develop bladder cancer than abstainers," says the *U.S. Pharmacist* report. A 1981 study suggested a link between caffeine and cancer of the pancreas, but that has not been confirmed in other studies.

Coffee is the major source of caffeine for most Americans. Just two cups a day can put you over "the safe limit," defined in this report as 200 milligrams. But did you know that a cup of drip or percolated coffee has nearly 80 milligrams of caffeine more than the same cup filled with instant coffee? If you don't like decaffeinated coffee (which contains five milligrams of caffeine), try instant coffee instead to cut your daily intake, the report suggests.

Some other caffeine counts to note are the following:

Brewed tea, 6 oz. cup — 50 milligrams of caffeine
Instant tea, 6 oz. cup — 30 milligrams
Cola drinks, 12 oz. — 30 to 50 milligrams
Hot cocoa, 6 oz. cup — 2 to 8 milligrams
Sweet, dark chocolate, 1 oz. — 5 to 35 milligrams
Chocolate desserts (ice cream, candy and puddings) — 10 milligrams

Note: Pain relief medication also can contain caffeine. One Excedrin tablet, for example, contains 65 milligrams of caffeine.

People who consume excess caffeine — 500 to 600 milligrams a day—might experience caffeinism, or "coffee nerves," and become addicted. You might be suffering from caffeinism if you have several symptoms like these: restlessness, insomnia, flushed face, stomach upset, nervousness and irregular heartbeat.

If you believe that you may be addicted, test yourself by not having your usual morning cup of coffee. If you have a severe headache later in the day, you likely have caffeinism. Such symptoms happen if you stop suddenly. Cutting back from large, daily doses of caffeine all at once might cause you to experience severe withdrawal symptoms, like throbbing headache, fatigue, irritability and anxiety.

Try to avoid "self-medicating" yourself with a cup of coffee. That's a step in the wrong direction, doctors say. Instead, try to cut down your caffeine habit gradually, rather than quitting "cold turkey." If you're drinking three cups of caffeinated coffee a day, try to cut back to two cups for a week or so. Then cut to one cup, and so forth.

Garbage-collecting HDL cholesterol helps heart

It seems everyone knows that too much cholesterol is bad for the heart. But a new study suggests that too little of a certain kind of cholesterol, high-density-lipoprotein cholesterol, can be equally bad for your health.

This "good" HDL acts like a vacuum cleaner in the bloodstream, sweeping up fatty cholesterol and preventing it from collecting on artery walls.

A large number of patients whose total cholesterol levels were considered "safe" had diseased heart arteries, the scientists reported. Current medical guidelines for cholesterol levels were issued in October 1987 by the National Cholesterol Education Program (NCEP).

This discovery about HDL levels has prompted the scientists to question whether the NCEP guidelines, used by most physicians in diagnosing patients, may need revision, according to *Medical World News* (29,23:26).

The researchers at the Johns Hopkins Medical Institutions in Baltimore evaluated the blood lipid (fat) content of 1,000 heart patients. These patients had undergone diagnostic coronary angiography, an X-ray of their heart arteries, to search for cholesterol-caused blockages of blood flow to the heart.

Of the 1,000 patients, there were 185 men and four, women who were found to have a combination of "safe" cholesterol levels and coronary artery disease. They were considered "safe" because their total cholesterol levels were less than 200, well within the so-called "desirable" range.

Patients in this group with a recent heart attack were excluded from the study because the heart attack would have altered their lipid levels. This left 138 men and three women in the investigation.

Sixty-eight percent of the men and 32 percent of the women had HDL-cholesterol levels of less than 35 milligrams per deciliter. Earlier studies have shown that the risk of heart disease increases as the HDL levels fall. An HDL level of 35 translates into a 50 percent higher risk than an HDL level of 45, according to the Framingham Heart Study.

The researchers "were curious to find out if, in fact, there were lipid abnormalities that were prevalent in a patient group that otherwise would not be detected by the present guidelines," said Dr. Michael Miller, one of the researchers. The guidelines, announced in 1987 by the National Cholesterol Education Program, define total cholesterol of less than 200 milligrams per deciliter (milligrams/dl) of blood as a desirable level for American adults.

Medical statistics show, and the Johns Hopkins study confirms, that a low HDL level is a strong predictor of coronary heart disease — even better, some scientists believe, than the presence of high levels of low-density lipoprotein (LDL).

Researchers say LDL contributes to coronary artery disease by depositing cholesterol on vessel walls. Scientists believe that HDL helps lower the risk of heart disease by transporting cholesterol to the liver to be processed for excretion. Therefore, low levels of HDL mean the blood doesn't have as many "garbage collectors" available to move out the cholesterol.

According to Miller, one way to increase HDL levels is to lose weight, particularly for obese patients. If you lose weight, not only will your HDL levels go up, but also your triglyceride levels might go down.

Most researchers think that high triglyceride levels in the blood also are a risk factor for heart disease.

In addition, weight loss reduces the risk of diabetes, which is itself a contributing factor to heart disease.

Exercising regularly and quitting smoking will also help to raise the good HDL levels.

Dietary changes commonly reduce blood cholesterol levels.

Polyunsaturated fats, such as those in corn or safflower oil, decrease total cholesterol levels, but they also lower HDL levels.

However, Miller says recent studies have shown that monounsaturated fats, such as olive oil, will reduce the total cholesterol without adversely affecting the HDL level.

Magnesium cuts risk of heart disease

Good news: if the drinking water in your area is considered "hard," that could be good news for your health! Hard water is rich in magnesium, and magnesium is a mineral that helps your nerves and muscles function properly.

Better news: scientists now realize that magnesium also plays a beneficial role in preventing heart disease. A new study described in *Science News* (137,14:214) suggests that magnesium teams up with a low-cholesterol diet to discourage atherosclerosis, or the buildup of fat deposits on the walls of coronary arteries.

Researchers believe that a good supply of magnesium in your diet discourages the production of cells that form the fatty deposits on artery walls.

Scientists also suggest that a diet that is too low in magnesium can cause your body to draw magnesium from your muscles. This reduces the amount of magnesium in the muscles that is necessary to keep the muscles working properly.

Unfortunately, magnesium alone will not prevent or cure atherosclerosis. Eating a low-cholesterol diet is still your best protection against this form of heart disease. However, you can strengthen your defenses by including high-magnesium foods in your menus.

Boost your body's supply of magnesium by eating more green vegetables, nuts, whole grains and shellfish — all good natural sources of this essential mineral. And as you protect your heart, you will also help your other muscles function smoothly.

Remember, check with your doctor before using vitamin supplements to increase your supply of magnesium.

'Miracle' clove reduces rates of heart attacks

For a long time, it seemed that garlic was popular with everybody except vampires and scientists.

For centuries, garlic has enjoyed great fame and popularity as a "miracle, cure-all" clove.

But scientists and researchers often dismissed the subject as simply another example of "primitive" folklore. Until now, that is.

Now, researchers are beginning to investigate the actual "powers" of garlic, and they like what they're finding.

Garlic seems to reduce the rates of heart attacks.

Garlic eaters had 32 percent fewer second heart attacks and 45 percent fewer deaths from heart attacks than non-garlic eaters, reports *Science News* (138,10:157).

Garlic also might interfere with the body's bad habit of over-producing cholesterol and other blood-clotting agents that contribute to heart disease, says *Science News*.

Another possible benefit of garlic compounds might be their "scavenging" effects.

Apparently, garlic increases the body's ability to remove substances in the blood that trigger cancer, says a recent study in *Preventive Medicine* (19,3: 346)

Garlic actually seems to "clean" the blood.

So, eating more garlic results in much lower rates of cancer, says the report.

For example, people in regions of China where average garlic consumption is high (a little less than one ounce per day) have lower rates of stomach cancer than people in the regions where the garlic intake is low.

The moral of the story? Add an extra bit of garlic to your diet.

It might be bad for your breath, but it could help save your life!

Olive oil gives double-barreled protection for your heart

Calling all cooks! Olive oil is good for more than tasty salads!

Studies show that olive oil provides double-barreled protection for your heart, reports the *Medical Tribune* (31,20:15).

Olive oil is rich in monounsaturated fatty acids, and these fatty acids can have two positive effects on your health.

1) Lowers cholesterol. Your doctor has been telling you to avoid saturated and hydrogenated fats (usually hardened fats, such as cooking lard) because they can raise your

cholesterol. However, olive oil is rich in unsaturated fats that can actually lower your LDL cholesterol level. (LDL cholesterol is the "bad" cholesterol.)

2) Reduces risk of atherosclerosis. This disease begins as "scratches" on the inside of your arteries. This is similar to rubbing coarse sandpaper on the inside of a plastic pipe. These "scratches" are a good place for cholesterol to attach and build up.

The scratches can be caused by a chemical change (oxidation) in the LDL cholesterol in your blood. The olive oil helps keep the chemical change in the LDL from happening. This reduces the chances of "scratches" forming and lowers your risk of heart disease.

So, stock your kitchen with olive oil. It's great in your salads, and it helps you protect a healthy heart!

Corny enough for you?

Olive oil may be great in your Greek salad and good for your heart, but corn oil might be even better for your heart's health.

Corn oil seems to be able to lower the level of plasma fibrinogen in the blood, reports the *Journal of the American College of Nutrition* (9,4:352).

Plasma fibrinogen is a kind of protein in the blood that helps make blood "sticky" and form clots. Too much fibrinogen causes the blood to "thicken" and clot abnormally.

Abnormal clotting is unhealthy and may contribute to strokes, atherosclerosis (hardening of the arteries) and heart disease.

Since some oils seem to lower the amount of fibrinogen, scientists wanted to find out which one does the best job: dietary fish oil, corn oil or olive oil.

They fed the oils to three groups of volunteers for eight weeks and then tallied the results.

The fish-oil group and the corn oil group were number one and two in lowering plasma fibrinogen. Olive oil was least effective and came in third.

Researchers already knew that fish oil lowers fibrinogen levels. But, what's new is the discovery that corn oil also does a good job in making blood more "slippery" and less liable to stick together in clots.

Corn oil might become the latest nutritional weapon against strokes and heart disease, the report suggests.

Fiber-up against heart attacks

Repeated studies have shown that fiber, especially "soluble" fiber like oat bran, can be extremely beneficial in helping to reduce the incidents of heart disease. You do not have to go into a scientific laboratory to see how a high-fiber diet has affected large numbers of people.

Around the turn of the century, heart attacks were relatively rare in this country. Now coronary heart disease is the number one killer in the U.S. Heart problems were also unknown or extremely rare among primitive people.

So many elements in our modern life seem to contribute directly to heart disease. Obesity, smoking, adding salt to foods, drinking soft water, drinking heavily chlorinated water, lack of exercise, not eating vegetable oils, eating saturated fats, eating sugar and other low-fiber foods and the hectic pace of modern life all have taken their toll on our nation's hearts.

Perhaps one of the most important factors has been our consumption of high-fat foods. This in turn has lead to an increase in blockage in blood vessels and other cardiovascular problems.

There are many reasons to believe that a high-fiber diet will reduce the likelihood of having a heart attack. Here are five:

- Low-fiber diets came into vogue about the same time that heart attacks started increasing.
- There is a close correlation in all areas of the world between the rate of diverticular disease, which is reduced by adding dietary fiber, and coronary heart disease.
- High-fiber diets help people to lose weight, and slim people have fewer heart attacks than those who are overweight.
- People on a high-fiber diet eliminate more cholesterol and have lower blood cholesterol levels than people on a low-fiber diet.
- Heart patients at the Pritikin Centers and other clinics have shown a remarkable improvement when placed on a diet containing mostly unrefined complex carbohydrates (starches that

contain natural fiber) plus regular exercise.

A little lean meat might not hurt your heart

A diet including lean meat might be "almost as effective" as a vegetarian diet in reducing your risk of heart disease, Australian researchers report in *The American Journal of Clinical Nutrition* (50,2:280). The real plus is this: more of us would stick to a diet that includes lean meat, the scientists believe.

In the study, 26 men from a fitness center ate one of three different diets—a high-fat "typical Australian" diet, a lean-meat diet, and a milk-egg-vegetable diet—for six-weeks so researchers could compare the risk-reduction benefits. The diets varied from 2,100 to 3,000 calories per day, based on individual needs as determined by metabolic tests. Only among the milk-egg-vegetable group was there a small loss of weight.

The researchers found that the milk-egg-veggie eaters cut their cholesterol levels by 10 percent. The lean-meat eaters cut their total cholesterol by 5 percent. Both "healthy" diets had a slight effect on blood pressure, lowering diastolic pressure an average of two to five points.

Participants on the lean-meat diet ate about nine ounces —slightly over a half-pound—of lean meat every day. The lean meat included combinations of processed ham, corned beef, chicken sausage, fresh beef and chicken. This lean-meat diet replaced 60 percent of the plant protein in the milk-egg-vegetable diet with meat protein.

Incidentally, the high-fat Australian diet was also high in cholesterol and low in fiber — similar to the typical American diet. Not surprisingly, men on this diet did not do as well as their counterparts on the other two diets.

During the study, researchers checked the participants' heart rate, blood pressure, and serum cholesterol levels every two weeks. They also checked high-density-lipoprotein (HDL or "good") cholesterol and low-density-lipoprotein (LDL or "bad") cholesterol levels.

Although men on the milk-egg-vegetable diet had the greatest reduction in blood pressure and cholesterol levels, the lean-meat diet "did not negate" the lowering of those two risk factors. Men on the high-fat diet had the least reduction, and, thus, the least benefit. However, the lean-meat diet also reduced "good" cholesterol, although researchers expected the reduction. They say the decline in HDL cholesterol would level off and stabilize over longer periods.

Researchers point out that in the milk-egg-vegetable diet, wheat — not soy — was the principal source of protein. In the current study, eating wheat protein led to an increase in glutamate, an amino acid relative that is linked to an excessive amount of cholesterol in the blood.

Although the lean-meat diet was less effective than the milk-egg-vegetable diet, researchers believe a diet including some lean meat is more acceptable to most people and would stand the best chance of long-term compliance.

A natural sugar that could harm your heart

If you're concerned about lowering your cholesterol levels and decreasing your heart attack risk, you should watch your fructose intake as well, researchers report in *The American Journal of Clinical Nutrition* (49,5:832). Fructose is a natural, simple sugar found in fruits and honey.

You get fructose another way, also. Your digestive system breaks down regular table sugar — sucrose — into about equal parts fructose and glucose. Of every 1,000 calories we eat and drink, about 100 calories — 10 percent — end up in the form of fructose, says a report on the study in *Science News* (133:196). Many doctors also recommend fructose as a partial replacement for regular sugar in their diets, *SN* says.

The researchers did a 10-week study to find out what would happen if the fructose intake were increased to 20 percent of a person's daily calories. For the first five weeks, the research team fed 21 men a typically American high-fat diet with the added fructose.

Some of the men in the test were found to have trouble regulating insulin and blood sugar levels. Those 12 with insulin-level problems were classified as hyperinsuline-mic. They had not been diagnosed before.

Each man consumed more than 3,200 calories a day on the non-weight-loss diet. The foods they ate exceeded limits of fat and cholesterol recommended by the American Heart Association. During the last five weeks, they replaced fructose with high-amylose cornstarch.

The fructose increased one heart-disease risk factor — uric acid levels — 13 percent among all participants. Although the increases in triglycerides and cholesterol "were small to moderate," researchers believe they signal a disturbing trend. That's because fructose is becoming a popular sweetener in many soft drinks and processed foods.

Perhaps the most ominous finding of the study was that "most cholesterol and triglyceride increases occurred in the very-low-density lipoproteins and low-density lipoproteins—the so-called 'bad' lipoproteins that increase the risk of heart disease," says the *Science News* report. People who already have high triglyceride levels are at highest risk. Ten of the 21 men in the study met this criterion.

In conclusion, a report in *The American Journal of Clinical Nutrition* (49,5:993) outlines how your diet can mean the difference between healthy maturity and lingering illnesses. Many studies concerning diet and your heart generally show that excess fat and sugar are risk factors for heart attack and artery disease.

One study examined diet and heart-disease deaths for 30 countries and found that fat, sugar, animal protein and total calories increased heart disease among men aged 55 to 59. Most experts recommend a balanced diet that cuts back on the amount of calories gotten from fat and cholesterol-containing foods. Cold-water fish provide a good source of omega-3 fatty acids, one kind of fat that seems to be good for your heart and circulatory system.

Starches and vegetable proteins are beneficial, according to the *Journal* report. Also, exercise more, and try to drop some weight, especially any "spare tire" of excess pounds around the middle.

CHAPTER 26

Heartburn

Heartburn alerts

For years, doctors have warned us not to mistake the warning symptoms of a heart attack for what they considered "harmless" heartburn.

Now, new studies suggest that heartburn itself might represent a real threat to your heart's health.

That burning or gnawing pain below the breastbone is triggered when stomach acid backs up into your esophagus, the food tube between the mouth and stomach.

We call it heartburn. Doctors call it gastroesophageal reflux.

A University of Maryland doctor reports that such acid back-ups actually can slow down the heartbeat by 20 beats a minute in otherwise healthy people.

Slowing down the heart rate could be dangerous for people with heart disease and previous heart attacks, says the report in *Geriatrics* (45,7:22).

Because of the risk involved with a slowed-down heart, doctors should be "aggressive" in treating reflux, especially among the elderly and people with heart-rhythm problems, says the report.

If you have heart disease and suffer regular episodes of heartburn, ask your doctor about this report in *Geriatrics*.

Your lungs also might be at risk.

That acid back-up into the esophagus might also trigger unexplained coughing and even asthma, says an editorial in *The Lancet* (336,8710:282).

About one out of every 10 chronic coughers could get relief by getting treatment for acid reflux, or heartburn, the article suggests.

A super-fine acid spray from the stomach possibly irritates lung and esophagus tissues, causing wheezing and asthmatic breathing spasms, the editorial says.

Some natural heartburn remedies include the following:

- Taking banana powder.
- Raising the head of your bed by six to eight inches.
- Avoiding food or drink for at least two hours before bedtime.
- Losing weight, especially around the middle.
- Sucking on candy-like lozenges (except peppermint-flavored ones).
- Eating more slowly, according to *New Natural Healing Encyclopedia* (FC&A, 1990: pg.193).

Check with your doctor about heartburn treatments.

CHAPTER 27

Immune System

Taking a 1,000-milligram tablet of vitamin C increases body temperature, quickly floods the bloodstream with the nutrient and seems to boost the immune system's resistance to infections.

So indicates an Arizona State University study in the *Journal of the American College of Nutrition* (9,2:150).

Turning up the heat is one way the body fights invading disease germs.

That heat rise triggered by the big dose might be why vitamin C seems to protect some people from the common cold, suggests researcher Carol S. Johnston.

In the study, healthy men and women took by mouth one daily tablet of the sodium ascorbate form of vitamin C, the equivalent of 17 times the RDA.

Besides raising their body temperatures, the big dose also lowered the concentration of iron in their blood.

While that sounds bad, it's actually not, since germs multiply more slowly with lowered iron levels.

The raised temperatures and lowered iron levels happened only when the people took that single, large, daily dose of vitamin C.

The same beneficial effects probably wouldn't happen if they simply took regular vitamin-mineral supplements every day, the report suggests.

That implies that you might be better off avoiding vitamin C in supplement form until you feel a cold or other infection coming on.

In any event, don't take supplements or megadoses of any nutrient without checking with your doctor first.

You can get the regular RDA of vitamin C in its natural form by eating at least two servings a day of citrus fruits, broccoli, brussels sprouts, strawberries, cantaloupe and dark-green, leafy vegetables.

CHAPTER 28

Insomnia

Seek sleepy relief with these:
* A glass of warm milk might be helpful. This is an old folk remedy that seems to have scientific basis to help insomnia. Dr. Ernest Hartmann in Boston has shown that L-tryptophan, an amino acid found abundantly in milk, helps people get to sleep easily. According to Dr. Hartmann's research, L-tryptophan stimulates the production of serotonin which is involved in the brain's sleep process. L-tryptophan supplements were once widely available in health food stores. A contaminated batch was linked to an outbreak of a crippling and sometimes deadly blood disease. Because L-tryptophan supplements might cause blood disorders and speed the aging process, you should stay away from the store-bought pills. Natural is still the best way to go. It seems that drinking warm milk is the best way to get the benefit of this amino acid. L-tryptophan

is also found in other dairy products, as well as in bananas, tuna, sardines (with bones), soybeans and turkey.

• Using hops, the flower of a grain used in flavoring beer, may help lull you to sleep, says Varro E. Tyler, Ph.D., dean of the schools of Pharmacy, Nursing and Health Sciences at Purdue University. Hops are known for their role in making beer, but they also have a sedative effect, he explains. But the sedative effect seems to come from sniffing the plant, not from drinking its by-product. A few years ago, people who harvested hops were found to become sleepy and tired after just a short time at work in the fields. Their behavior led to the discovery of hops as a sedative, according to Dr. Tyler. For the best sedative effect, Dr. Tyler suggests putting some hops in a muslin or cloth bag and using the bag as a pillow.

• Eat carbohydrates at your evening meal or as the last food you eat before going to bed. Eating meals composed mainly of carbohydrates might help people relax and feel drowsy, according to research at Texas Tech University. Psychology professor Dr. Bonnie Spring measured the difference between the effects of carbohydrate and protein meals in 184 people. Proteins made the people feel tense, but carbohydrates relaxed the men and made the women feel drowsy.

• Try "white noise." That's a soothing sound

produced by a fan or humidifier motor. There also are electronic makers of "white noise" that produce sounds like falling rain and waterfalls. The "white noise" masks other distracting noises, allowing many people to fall asleep quickly. Other possibilities are cassette tapes of ocean surf and other natural sounds.

Things to avoid:
- Caffeine. Avoid all sources including coffee, tea, chocolate, soft drinks, diet pills and some prescriptions and over-the-counter drugs. Ask your pharmacist for a complete list of drugs that contain caffeine.

CHAPTER 29

Kidneys and Urinary Tract Health

Rice fights kidney stones

Rice bran might help lower your risk of developing calcium-containing urinary stones. It does that by decreasing the amount of calcium excreted in the urine, reports the *Journal of Urology* (132:1140-5).

"In almost all patients, rice bran caused a significant decrease in urinary calcium excretion," wrote Dr. Ohkawa, one of the researchers. "Evidence of stones has decreased clearly among patients treated with rice bran for one to three years....We suggest that...rice bran treatment should be effective for prevention of recurrent urinary stone disease."

The *British Journal of Urology* (58:592-5) also reported rice bran's ability to limit urinary calcium and stone production.

Cranberry juice might be a weapon against urinary infections

Does cranberry juice prevent or fight urinary tract

infections? Several clinical studies suggest that drinking the sweetened juice of the otherwise bitter berry may cause two changes in the body. The two beneficial changes help in the fight against infections in the pipeline from the kidneys through the bladder.

In one study, reported in *U.S. Pharmacist* (14,5:35), 60 people with urinary infections drank a pint of cranberry juice each day for 21 days. Otherwise, they took no special medications. More than half showed a significant improvement. Two out of 10 were slightly better, and about three out of 10 showed no improvement. In addition, six weeks after they all stopped drinking the juice, more than half who showed some improvement came down with another urinary infection.

Two other studies reported in the journal also showed some benefits after people drank the juice.

Researchers think cranberry juice raises the acid level of urine, causing it to become hostile to germs. They also think the fructose (a kind of sugar) used to sweeten the juice somehow makes mucous tissue inside the urinary system "slippery" to bacteria — the germs can't grab onto body tissue and multiply.

CHAPTER 30

Longevity

Can vitamins delay old age?

Can vitamin supplements actually help improve the immune system and delay the aging process? Scientists now think it might be possible.

Vitamin supplements might help strengthen the immune system in elderly people, suggests a study in *The Journal of the American College of Nutrition* (9,4:363).

Maintaining a proper balance and amount of vitamins is crucial in helping the body ward off illnesses quickly and effectively. However, the study shows that most elderly people frequently have low levels of important vitamins in their bodies.

Unfortunately, this shortage of important vitamins often results in a sluggish immune system that has great trouble fighting off sicknesses. So, many elderly people suffer needlessly from common illnesses simply because their immune systems have slowed down.

Many elderly people eat very well-balanced meals, but they still suffer from vitamin deficiencies. This is because the other medications they take often block the vitamins in the food from being absorbed and used in the body.

So, scientists are suggesting that elderly people talk to their physicians about vitamin supplements to help bring the amount of vitamins in the body up to the proper level and help the immune system function as effectively as possible.

Eat less, live longer

Saying "no thanks" to seconds at the dinner table might actually help prolong your life, Texas researchers report in *Geriatrics* (44:12,87).

Reducing calories prolonged the lives of healthy rats in their study, but did not stunt growth, researchers said. Even animals with heart and kidney problems lived longer and developed tumors later in life than rats on unrestricted diets.

The rats on restricted diets lived longer than those who ate freely, researchers said.

Other benefits of a disciplined diet include healthier bones and improved immunity, they added.

Would humans reap similar benefits? Scientists have known for some time that diet, growth and aging are related, but animal studies such as this are the first step in understanding how diet might prolong human life.

Researchers have several theories. This study suggests that digesting three well-balanced meals a day constitutes an eight-hour workday for your body. Eating more than you need means your cells must work overtime to digest the extra food.

"Tired" cells weaken with age and can't fight disease and illness effectively. In a nutshell, the less you eat, the less work for your body.

What you eat might also be a significant factor in prolonging life, researchers said. Chemicals in certain foods cause a "red alert" in your body, meaning that it must work double-overtime to digest them.

Further studies will look at what foods cause this response in the body.

In the meantime, eating less seems to have many more positive benefits than always eating until you're stuffed.

CHAPTER 31

Memory and Mind Problems

Can vitamins and mineral supplements make you smarter?

We've often been told that we "are what we eat," but a new study takes that a step further. It suggests that our intelligence level may be linked to adequate amounts of vitamins and minerals.

In just one school year, tests on 90 high school students in Britain showed an increase in IQ scores in children taking nutritional supplements. Children taking a placebo (a harmless, fake drug) and children not taking anything were used for comparison. Yet, the children receiving the supplements had a marked difference in their non-verbal IQ scores, according to *The Lancet*, a British medical journal.

Nutritionists know which vitamins and minerals aid development in different parts of our brain and body. Yet most believed that people in Western countries received adequate amounts of the necessary vitamins and minerals through their everyday diet.

This is the first study that has been able to document

changes in intelligence based on vitamin and mineral supplementation in people who were not technically deficient. David Benton, who conducted the study, considers the results preliminary. But if you want to start taking more vitamins and minerals, you should use supplements that contain them in the ratios set by the U.S. government and known as the Recommended Dietary Allowance (RDA).

Supplements to counteract senility

Senility is memory loss, disorientation, confusion and loss of reasoning ability with advancing age. There is a difference between the natural slowing of our reaction time with advancing age and being senile. Only a small percentage of older Americans suffer from true senility.

Good nutrition and other practices that promote good health may help prevent senility.

Pantothenic acid (vitamin B5) supplements may improve symptoms of senility and depression when taken with other B vitamins.

Confusion might mean a nutritional deficiency

It's considered a medical emergency. Doctors see signs of mental confusion, verbal nonsense, wobbly walk, uncoordinated movements and eyesight disturbances in people with a severe deficiency of vitamin B1, also called thiamine.

"The age-old and potentially fatal nutritional deficiency... requires immediate thiamine (B1) replacement to ensure the best long-term outcome," says an article in *Emergency Medicine* (21,7:13). "Withholding treatment for only a few hours from patients you may think have the disease may worsen the prognosis."

The condition, known medically as Wernicke's encephalopathy, can strike not only alcoholics but also people with kidney disease, patients with thyroid gland problems, and compulsive dieters suffering from self-induced starvation, a condition called anorexia nervosa.

While its symptoms are serious, the disease itself "is probably totally reversible if treated early," the report said. Even a previously healthy person can drain her body's entire supply of thiamine within three weeks, the report warns. That's especially true if the person is for any reason receiving an intravenous infusion of glucose over a period of several days.

Thiamine is a water-soluble vitamin, the first of the B vitamins to be isolated in its pure form (that's why it's known as B1). Normal levels of thiamine are necessary for converting carbohydrates in food into energy, for the proper operation of the nervous system, and for growth and repair of body tissues. Thiamine is found naturally in yeast, liver, whole-grain products, wheat, eggs, milk, nuts, potatoes, leafy green vegetables, kidney beans, and seeds.

"The need for thiamine is increased when carbohydrate consumption is high," according to *Vitamin and Mineral Encyclopedia* (FC&A Publishing, 1987: p. 92). Exercise or emotional stress may increase the energy needs of the body and the body's need for thiamine. More thiamine is needed in pregnancy, during breast-feeding, when fever is present, during and after surgery, and in cases of hyperthyroidism.

Other things that deplete thiamine include sulfa drugs, oral contraceptives and estrogen hormone treatments, air pollution and certain food additives like nitrates and sulfates.

Men over 50 normally need about 1.2 milligrams of thiamine each day. Adult women need somewhat less, about 1 milligram. However, if special conditions warrant, your regular thiamine intake may need to be supplemented.

Always be sure to ask your doctor or healthcare provider about supplements, however, because certain people should not take thiamine. In diabetics, for example, thiamine supplements can interfere with insulin levels in the blood.

Senile? It might only be a nutrient you're missing

Senile dementia, which manifests itself in mental failure, is thought to be genetically based, according to *The Lancet*. That prognosis does not leave those afflicted with it much hope.

To deal with a genetically-based disorder requires some medical way of modifying or blocking a chemical process, *The Lancet* reports.

Based on research and examination of other genetically-based diseases, Burnet believes the root of dementia may be a simple lack of an important nutrient: zinc. Burnet cites the congenital childhood disease acrodermatitis enteropathica as an example of zinc's effectiveness on genetically-based disorders. Zinc supplements remove the accompanying symptoms of skin rash and diarrhea. Since infants with acrodermatitis enteropathica often take in enough zinc in their diets, Burnet speculates the disease is caused by "some genetic anomaly in the absorption or utilization of the available zinc." It is reasonable to suggest, he adds, that genetic-based zinc deficiency may be relatively common.

Dementia basically involves a loss of neurons (nerve cells), Burnet says. He believes neurons die because of some genetic error within them, which, because of age, causes loss of ability to make zinc available.

While cell death is normal as we age, the "devastating fallout of neurons in dementia," Burnet thinks, is due to lack of zinc.

Although more research should be done to confirm his idea, Burnet believes zinc supplements might be the answer for many dementia patients. The recommended daily dietary allowance of zinc for adults is 15 milligrams per day.

Burnet's opinion is reinforced by a British doctor, Roy Hullin, who found lower levels of zinc in people who were senile than in people who were not senile. Dr. Hullin feels that the elderly do not get enough zinc in their diets. Zinc is plentiful in meats and seafood.

CHAPTER 32

Osteoporosis and Bone Health

Osteoporosis — the brittle-bone disease — is an equal-opportunity illness, affecting both women and men, new research suggests.

Latest finding: men in later life lose about 2.3 percent of spinal bone every year, reports a study in *Annals of Internal Medicine* (112:1:29).

Men from age 30 on lose about 1 percent per year of bone mass in the wrists and hands, the study says.

The rate of bone loss in the hands and wrists gets worse as men get older, the study says.

Until now, most researchers thought osteoporosis affected mainly women past menopause.

For that reason, nutritionists recently boosted the Recommended Dietary Allowance (RDA) of calcium for younger women, believing more calcium at a younger age may help prevent brittle bones in later years.

Now, they might have to rethink the RDA for younger men as well.

Unfortunately, the study also suggested that taking calcium supplements later in life seemed not to stop or even to slow the rate of bone loss in men.

"We found a substantial rate of bone loss, despite a generous calcium intake," the study reports.

The abnormal amount of bone loss is the result of calcium in the bones being drawn out into the blood and excreted in the urine. The bones become brittle, the amount of bone mass is reduced, and the strength of remaining bone is weakened.

Osteoporosis causes the stooped posture and distinctive "dowager's hump" in elderly women. It usually begins to show up in women past the menopause.

It's also responsible for many of the hip, leg and arm fractures suffered by many older people, the report says.

Take steps to prevent osteoporosis

The best way to manage osteoporosis is to prevent it from developing. Since osteoporosis develops silently over many years, proper diet and exercise, throughout your life, are extremely important.

- Adequate calcium. The daily diet should include foods that are high in calcium like dairy products (including milk, cheese, and yogurt), dark-green, leafy vegetables (like collards, turnip greens, spinach and broccoli), salmon, sardines, oysters, and tofu.

- Adequate vitamin D. Vitamin-fortified milk, cereals, saltwater fish, liver and daily sunshine are good sources of this vitamin.

- Adequate manganese. Manganese is an important mineral found in whole-grain products, fruits (especially bananas), vegetables (especially legumes), eggs, liver and other organ meats.

• Adequate exercise. Walking, jogging, dancing, bicycling, aerobics, rowing, hiking, rope jumping, tennis and other exercise in which the bones have to support body weight, helps promote bone growth.

• With your doctor, consider estrogen replacement therapy during menopause. When estrogen replacement therapy is started right after women stop menstruating, hip and wrist fractures can be reduced as much as 60 percent.

• Avoid smoking, alcoholic beverages, drinks containing caffeine, soft drinks, meat, and high-protein foods.

Source: National Institutes of Health and *Stand Tall* by Notelovitz and Ware.

Antacids that affect your bones

You were probably thinking of your stomach and not your bones when you took that antacid. However, antacids have ingredients that can make a big difference to the health of your bones.

Avoid antacids that contain aluminum. Aluminum draws phosphorus out of the bones and makes the body more susceptible to osteoporosis. Antacids containing aluminum include: Camalox, Delcid, Di-Gel, Gaviscon, Gelusil-M, Gelusil-II, Maalox, Maalox Plus, Nephrox, Tempo, WinGel, ALternaGEL, Aludrox, Amphojel, Mylanta, Mylanta-II, and Simeco. Large amounts of these taken over long periods of time may be very harmful to your bones.

Antacids like Tums, which have only calcium carbonate as an active ingredient, actually have a protective effect — they provide calcium necessary for healthy bones and prevention of osteoporosis. Although Tums and some other antacids contain calcium, some doctors do not recommend using antacids for a daily calcium supplement because in large quantities they may aggravate your digestive system and cause constipation.

How caffeine affects your bones

To prevent osteoporosis, we have to guard against calcium being leached out of our bones. Several studies have shown the negative effect of coffee in causing bone loss. But new research has just confirmed that it is the caffeine in coffee that causes calcium loss. Put simply, the more caffeine you drink, the more calcium is driven out of your bones.

At Mt. Saint Vincent University in Halifax, Nova Scotia, researcher Susan Whiting tested different properties of coffee in animals to determine exactly what causes the loss of calcium. Whiting demonstrated that it is the caffeine in coffee, not the diuretic effect, that takes calcium from the body.

In another study, Dr. Linda K. Massey reported that caffeinated-coffee drinkers lose twice as much calcium as people who drink decaffeinated coffee. In her work at Washington State University, Massey found that caffeine causes calcium to be excreted in urine.

Since many coffee drinkers are not getting enough calcium to begin with, drinking coffee containing caffeine is making their problem worse, Massey believes.

People who drink large amounts of caffeinated beverages, including tea and some cola drinks, may have an increased risk of osteoporosis, reports *Science News* (138,16:253).

Researchers suggest that people who drink two to three cups of caffeinated coffee daily, or five to six cups of caffeinated tea daily, have almost a 70-percent greater risk of osteoporosis than those people who do not drink caffeine.

And people who drink three to four cups of coffee daily or six to seven cups of tea daily seem to have an 82-percent increased risk of osteoporosis compared to people who do not drink caffeinated beverages.

Apparently, the caffeine prevents the digestive system from absorbing enough calcium from the diet, and caffeine increases the amount of calcium that is lost in the urine.

The decreased amount of calcium in the body can result in osteoporosis.

So, if you drink caffeinated drinks, make sure you keep the number of cups each day below a safe level. Smoking and drinking too much alcohol can also increase your risk of developing osteoporosis.

Study says calcium needed throughout life

To get the best protection against osteoporosis, you should make sure you get the recommended amounts of calcium in your diet beginning early in life, a new study revealed in the *Journal of the American Medical Association* (260:3150-55).

Women with high-calcium diets throughout their lives, as children, adolescents, and reproductive women, have the highest bone density, according to the study. "Swallowing calcium pills at 50 years of age probably is not going to make your bones thicker," Kuller said.

"In our analysis, the only group in which a protective effect of calcium could be observed was in women who reported both a high milk consumption during periods of growth and development, as well as currently," the report concluded.

Damage from osteoporosis is usually permanent. The most common treatments include heat, drugs for the pain, a back brace and rest. Rest, combined with moderate exercise like walking, helps keep the muscles in shape to support the weak bone structure. Since damage from osteoporosis is difficult to repair, prevention should be a life-long goal.

Too much salt causes body to lose calcium

Too much salt in the diet may increase a woman's chances of suffering osteoporosis after menopause, Canadian researchers report in *The American Journal of Clinical Nutrition* (50,5:1088).

They studied 17 women aged 52 to 72 who ate their usual diet and were then given salt supplements.

Excess salt causes the body to rid itself of calcium through urination, researchers say. Many postmenopausal women do not get enough calcium to begin with, they add

If salt intake is low, women susceptible to osteoporosis might need less calcium after menopause, a New Zealand team of researchers concludes in the *British Medical Journal* (299,6703:834).

Thus, if you eat less salt, you might enjoy better bone health, the study suggests.

Ten women over age 65 volunteered for the study. They alternated their regular diet with low-salt and high-salt diets for periods of 10 days.

Women on the low-salt diet had the least loss of calcium, followed by the regular diet and high-salt diet groups.

Osteoporosis is a crippling bone disease that strikes mostly among women over 50.

Vitamin D helps fight crippling bone loss

If you have passed menopause and want to protect yourself from osteoporosis, be careful not to neglect your vitamin D. According to a report in *The New England Journal of Medicine* (321,26:1777), vitamin D is an important weapon in fighting crippling bone loss.

Without proper amounts of vitamin D, your body cannot regulate the level of parathyroid hormones that it makes. Parathyroid hormones can speed up bone loss by interfering with the body's absorption of calcium.

It's true that calcium is a major building block of strong bones, but you can't eat enough foods rich in calcium to make up for a diet low in vitamin D. When vitamin D levels drop, too many parathyroid hormones are produced.

When this happens, the body loses its ability to use the extra calcium.

In other words, you may be eating a lot of calcium, but your body can't use it because you don't have enough vitamin D.

Unless vitamin D levels are increased, you still run the risk of harmful bone loss, even with added calcium.

Researchers stress the importance of getting enough vitamin D in the diet, especially when exposure to sunlight is limited.

Your body produces vitamin D naturally in sunlight, enabling the body to keep parathyroid hormones below dangerous levels.

Vitamin D supplements during winter months help maintain hormone levels that would ordinarily vary from summer to winter. Without the advantage of vitamin D supplements, many women experience seasonal bone loss.

The report also states there is no evidence that an intake of vitamin D sufficient to protect you in winter would be intolerable during warm-weather exposure to the sun.

Fluoride fails to prevent osteoporosis

Thinner, weaker bones trouble many women in the years after menopause. In other countries, doctors have widely recommended sodium fluoride as a treatment for this condition. But, according to the *Mayo Clinic Health Letter* (8,4:5), new bone growth stimulated by sodium fluoride is so weak that it actually fractures more easily.

The best way to strengthen your bones is to exercise regularly and eat a diet rich in calcium-containing foods like dark-green vegetables, dairy products and canned salmon or sardines.

Careful where you get your calcium

Calcium supplements containing bone meal often contain lead, and large doses of the bone meal could cause lead poisoning, scientists from the University of Illinois warn.

Many women use large daily doses of bone meal as a calcium supplement, since it is cheaper than most other sources of calcium. However, bone meal is not technically a drug or food, so the labeling and quality control for it is not as stringent as it is for regular calcium supplements.

OJ helps prevent bone loss

When you have breakfast, make sure you don't leave out a glass of orange juice. You could be depriving your body of its most easily absorbed source of calcium, in the form of calcium-enriched orange juice.

Calcium-fortified orange juice contains a form of calcium known as calcium citrate malate. This form of calcium is readily absorbed and used by the body. Calcium citrate malate is especially helpful in preventing bone loss from the spine, reports *The New England Journal of Medicine* (323,13:878).

Talk with your doctor about adding calcium-fortified orange juice to your diet. The convenience of calcium-enriched orange juice is a refreshing way to increase your daily intake of calcium while quenching your thirst.

CHAPTER 33

Premenstrual Syndrome (PMS)

Relief from PMS

Don't suffer the monthly terrors of PMS (premenstrual syndrome) without a fight. Here are some useful weapons:

- Vitamin B6 (pyridoxine) can be taken daily in premenstrual times. It helps relieve fluid retention, weight gain, arthritis associated with female hormone deficiency, and symptoms of depression.
- Supplements of the amino acid DLPA (d,l, phenylalanine) provide amazing relief to chronic PMS sufferers, according to current research. This amino acid has been found to be the substance in chocolate that causes many people to crave chocolate. For maximum effectiveness, supplements should be taken daily at mealtimes for several weeks.
- Avoid coffee and caffeine. The more coffee you drink, the more severe your PMS symptoms usually become (*Amer-*

ican Journal of Public Health 75: 11, 1135).

Women with the most severe PMS problems were found to drink four or more cups of coffee daily. Despite this discovery, many over-the-counter products for PMS contain caffeine; so remember to read the labels.

Check with your doctor before taking supplements.

CHAPTER 34

Skin Problems

Preventing purple age spots

Are frequent bruises and those dark purple spots that appear in old age inevitable? No, according to Dr. Oscar Gyde, a British hematologist.

A test of 20 elderly patients with age spots and 20 without at England's Fast Birmingham Hospital revealed that besides the age spots "the only measurable difference between the two groups was the level of zinc in their body," Gyde says. "The elderly without the spots on their skin had a higher level of zinc. The elderly with spots had a significantly lower level of zinc," says Gyde.

Dr. Gyde concluded from the study that age spots "are not simply an unsightly sign of aging. Their presence means you should suspect a zinc deficiency."

The purple spots, not to be confused with brown age spots, occur when the tiny blood vessels in the skin rupture and bleed. They eventually disappear on their own, Gyde explains.

"The role of zinc would be to prevent them from

appearing in the first place or from reappearing," he says.

Dr. Mary Dundas of the University of Tennessee advises eating foods high in zinc as a preventive measure. Those foods include such high protein fares as shellfish, oysters, red meat and liver.

You may also want to check with your doctor about zinc supplements, Dr. Gyde adds. The recommended daily dietary allowance of zinc for adults is 15 milligrams per day for men over 50 and 12 milligrams for women.

The brown age spots that often appear later in life may be helped by pantothenic acid, vitamin B5. A biology professor at Mary Washington College in Virginia, Thomas L. Johnson, Ph.D., contends that daily supplements of pantothenic acid completely cleared brown age spots in just a few months.

However, be careful when considering vitamin-B5 supplements. These supplements can change the action of high blood-pressure and blood-thinning drugs. Pantothenic acid may also increase premature skin wrinkles in people who smoke. Pantothenic acid is found naturally in yeast, whole-grain products, liver, salmon, eggs, beans, seeds, peanuts, mushrooms, elderberries and citrus fruit.

The best way to prevent the brown age spots is by avoiding exposure to the sun and sunlamps.

Avoid alcohol if you suffer from psoriasis

A high alcohol intake worsens psoriasis, Finnish researchers report in the *British Medical Journal* (300,6727:780).

For two years, they studied 429 men (144 with psoriasis and 285 with other skin diseases) aged 19 to 50 and asked them the following questions:

- Does drinking increase the risk of psoriasis?
- Does drinking worsen psoriasis?
- Does psoriasis increase drinking?

Participants filled out a questionnaire about their drinking habits the year before their skin disease developed and the year before they joined the study.

Psoriasis was not associated with any other factor, such as age, social class or marital status.

"Alcohol intake and frequency of intoxication were individually the only significant explaining variables," researchers said.

Also, psoriasis patients reported that their drinking had increased after the disease was diagnosed, and one third reported that alcohol seemed to worsen their psoriasis.

Those who had psoriasis on a greater portion of their body tended to drink more as well.

Those findings lead researchers to suggest that psoriasis "sustains" drinking in some patients.

Vitamin D cream for psoriasis

People with the dry, scaly skin disease known as psoriasis might find relief by using a skin cream containing an active form of vitamin D, according to a digest in *American*

Family Physician (40,4:301).

More than three out of four psoriasis sufferers got consistent relief by applying calcitriol in a petroleum jelly base to the scaly areas.

Most got better without any side effects from the vitamin. Calcitriol is known medically as vitamin D3.

Dr. Michael F. Holick, the director of the Vitamin D, Skin and Bone Research Laboratory at Boston City Hospital, also is excited about his latest research on psoriasis.

His researchers have found that an "active form of vitamin D is able to inhibit the growth of skin cells" which cause psoriasis, he says.

Until now, no treatment for the scaly, itchy skin of psoriasis has been completely effective or free of side effects, *Prevention* magazine reports.

The results of Dr. Holick's research, published in the *Archives of Dermatology*, offer the most promising news for psoriasis sufferers yet.

"Sixty percent of our patients respond to this therapy," Holick says. Redness and scales on the scalp have decreased markedly, and their lesions eventually cleared up.

Further research on 200 psoriasis patients was scheduled to make sure there are no side effects to the drug.

Holick notes that store-bought vitamin D will be "of no use for treating psoriasis," and that, taken in large doses, it can be toxic. For right now, the psoriasis-fighting form of vitamin D is available only in Holick's study.

For psoriasis sufferers, approval of the new drug will be a welcome relief.

Vitamin A looks promising

Derivatives of vitamin A are used as prescription treatments for acne. So, although vitamin A is not routinely given for psoriasis, it is known to help the skin. Vitamin A maintains the smoothness, health and functioning of the skin and the mucous membranes. Vitamin A also helps build body protein and promotes the growth of body tissues.

However, large doses of vitamin A can cause severe side effects. So doctors warn against taking more than the RDA (Recommended Dietary Allowance)—5 micrograms daily for men and women over 50. You can get vitamin A naturally by eating healthy amounts of fruits and vegetables, particularly yellow vegetables like carrots and squash. You can also get vitamin A by eating liver or taking cod liver oil.

Skin ulcers

In tests in hospital patients, people with healing problems like leg ulcers or pressure sores also had the lowest levels of zinc in their bodies, reports *The British Journal of Nutrition* (59,2:181).

Higher levels of zinc might help your skin heal faster, the report suggests.

Avoid these 'juicy fruits'

Photosensitivity is an exaggerated reaction to sunlight.

It can be caused by using certain drugs, cosmetics, or perfumes, according to *Patient Care* (6:15). Redness, swelling, hives and itching are symptoms of photosensitivity. If your skin is photosensitive, it reacts to the sun more quickly and more severely than normal skin.

Even eating some foods can bring a reaction. Limes, celery, lemons, parsley, and certain oranges can cause photosensitivity, Dr. Jonathan Held reports in the *American Family Physician* (39,4:143).

If the skin is exposed to one of these fruits or vegetables and then the ultraviolet rays of the sun, a severe skin irritation may occur. The irritation may take the form of redness, itching and rash. Redness and blistering usually appear about 48 hours after exposure.

Grocery workers are especially vulnerable to this type of skin irritation. They should be careful to avoid direct contact with limes, celery, lemons, parsley and bergamot oranges.

CHAPTER 35

Strokes

The nutrient that cuts the risk of fatal stroke by nearly half

There's an easy way to slash your risk of having a fatal stroke — eat one extra serving of fresh fruit or vegetables every day, declares a major dietary study. The super stroke preventer is the nutrient potassium, abundant in fresh fruits and vegetables, according to doctors Kay-Tee Khaw and Elizabeth Barrett-Connor and reported in *Medical World News* (30,11:30).

These researchers raised the possibility of potassium being a stroke fighter in a big study in 1987. Since then, three separate medical studies have demonstrated that increased potassium in the diet can dramatically lower your risk of death from stroke, the report says.

The studies found that groups of people that ate the most fruits and vegetables had 25 to 40 percent fewer fatal strokes than groups with lower potassium intakes. According to the report, women benefited from a high-potassium diet even more than men. The people in the studies all were

59 or older.

"Americans could raise their potassium levels significantly by simply cutting down on junk food and substituting orange or grapefruit juice for soft drinks," according to the report.

Blood vessel disease — 'B'-ware!

If your doctor has warned you about your risk of strokes or blood vessel diseases, but you're not suffering from high cholesterol levels, vitamin B may be just what you need.

The American Heart Association reports that a metabolic defect that can lead to blood vessel disease and increase the risk of stroke may be corrected with vitamin-B supplements.

The defect is known as "mild hyperhomocysteinemia." This condition results in slight to moderate elevations of homocysteine, an amino acid that circulates in the blood.

At normal levels, this amino acid is harmless. But research indicates that mildly elevated levels might damage blood vessels and possibly lead to atherosclerosis or "hardening of the arteries."

The American Heart Association reports that excess homocysteine seems to damage blood vessels. Homocysteine causes sores and scars to form on blood vessel walls, similar to how cholesterol does.

If a blood clot forms on the lesions and blocks blood flow to the heart or brain, it can trigger a heart attack or stroke.

The good news is that vitamin B can help break down

extra homocysteine in the blood and prevent dangerous buildups of the amino acid.

B vitamins (biotin, B6, B12) convert the homocysteine to a harmless kind of amino acid called methionine.

Eliminating the extra homocysteine from the blood greatly reduces the risk of blood vessel diseases.

People who have suffered from hardening of the arteries that could not be explained by high cholesterol levels are the most likely suspects for mild hyperhomocysteinemia.

But don't try to treat yourself without your doctor's advice!

If you're concerned about your risk of blood vessel disease, talk to your doctor about the best type of therapy for you.

C for softer arteries

A new role for vitamin C might be in fighting cholesterol plaque buildup in arteries, suggests a study reported in the *Medical Tribune* (31,16:14).

Vitamin C stays on the job far longer than vitamin E in fighting oxidation of low-density lipoprotein (the "bad" LDL form of cholesterol).

University of Texas researchers believe oxidized LDL triggers atherosclerosis, or hardening of the arteries.

Because vitamin C does such a good job of battling this cholesterol, Dr. Ishwarlal Jialal suggests that the RDA should be doubled, from 60 milligrams to 120, the article says.

Hardening of the arteries causes heart disease and some strokes.

Vitamin C's best-known prevention role probably is its ability to neutralize several cancer-causing chemicals in cooked and processed foods.

It also acts as an antioxidant against so-called free radicals, tissue-harming substances brought into the bloodstream by food, air pollution and tobacco smoke.

Vitamin E helps reverse damage from hardening of the arteries

If you're suffering from atherosclerosis, or you have a family history of atherosclerosis (hardening of the arteries) and you fear that you might develop it, vitamin E might be the vitamin for you.

Vitamin E is taking a leading role in the fight against atherosclerosis, reports a recent digest in *Nutrition Today* (25,5:5).

Based on recent studies, vitamin E seems to help prevent the development of atherosclerosis, and it also seems to help reduce the damage if atherosclerosis has already begun.

The study reports that lab animals that were fed diets without vitamin E had about 79 percent more artery blockage than those animals fed the same diet but containing vitamin E.

Researchers also fed vitamin-E-enriched diets to lab animals that had been suffering from atherosclerosis for at least one year. After two years on a diet rich in vitamin E, the animals went from having 35 percent artery blockage to 15 percent.

The protective factor might lie in the vitamin's ability to clean up the blood, says a report in the *Medical Tribune* (31,19:11).

Vitamin E works as an "antioxidant" in the cells of your body. This means that it prevents oxygen molecules from combining with parts of the cell that would result in dangerous products.

For example, LDL cholesterol molecules occasionally combine with oxygen molecules to create "oxidized LDLs." These oxidized LDLs seem to damage cells, and scientists suspect that they might be one of the root causes of atherosclerosis.

Vitamin E functions as an antioxidant and prevents the LDLs from becoming oxidized. This protects the cells from damage and helps prevent atherosclerosis.

Researchers suggest that dietary antioxidants such as vitamin E could be a vital part of the treatment strategies for people with atherosclerosis as well as a good protection device for people seeking to avoid the disease.

Large amounts of vitamin E can be harmful, so never take vitamin-E supplements without first talking to your doctor.

Salt causes brain damage?

Too much salt in your diet may be harmful to more than

just your blood pressure.

According to *Science News* (137,15:238), researchers think that salt might cause brain tissue damage.

Apparently, too much salt in the diet damages and narrows artery walls.

These narrow arteries cut off blood supplies to the brain, which results in brain tissue damage and could lead to a stroke.

Maintaining a low-salt diet can decrease the risk of brain tissue damage.

CHAPTER 36

Teeth and Gum Health

Homemade toothpaste
prevents gum disease

If you are bothered by gum disease or pyorrhea, you might want to make your own dentifrice from a simple salt solution.

Dr. Paul Keyes, who has done work at the National Institute of Dental Research, states that he has never seen a case of gum disease in a person who has regularly used salt or a soda dentifrice. He advocates brushing with a solution made by putting water in a glass and pouring enough salt in it so that no more will dissolve after stirring. Dr. Keyes says that his program is also good for treating early stages of pyorrhea.

Other dentists recommend brushing with baking soda. It also has a scouring effect that helps clean the gum line where gum disease and decay start around plaque that forms there. Be careful when following this advice. Excessive scouring can wear away tooth enamel and cause pain when drinking acidic beverages.

These natural cleansers may be just what the doctor ordered to help you keep your teeth. Check with your dentist about the best care for your teeth and gums.

CHAPTER 37

Vision Problems

Natural ways to prevent cataracts

Cataracts occur when the lens of the eye becomes cloudy, often with advancing age. It might start when an enzyme system, which helps keep the lens of the eye clear, performs less efficiently with age. Factors contributing to the development of cataracts are:

•Exposure to ultraviolet light. Wearing sunglasses in bright sunlight or avoiding bright sunlight may be helpful in preventing cataracts.

•Riboflavin (vitamin B2) deficiency might be one cause of cataracts. There are reports of cataracts diminishing after supplements of riboflavin were taken, but these claims are unconfirmed at this time. On the other hand, taking large doses of the vitamin niacin (vitamin B3) or other B vitamins might increase the chances of getting cataracts.

Additional vitamin C has been found to lower the risk of cataracts, according to a study at Tufts University by Allan Taylor, M.D. Vitamin C seems to stop cataracts by blocking the proteins that form cataracts on the lens of the eye. High amounts of vitamin C are naturally found in uncooked rose hips, acerola cherries, citrus fruits, green peppers, parsley, broccoli, brussels sprouts, cabbage and potatoes.

Prevent cataracts naturally

People who take regular daily doses of either vitamin C or vitamin E might slash by more than half their risk of developing blinding cataracts, a new scientific study suggests. Those results come from a Canadian study of 175 cataract patients and 175 people without cataracts, according to a report in *Science News* (135,20:308). All those studied were over age 55.

"The scientists found that the only significant difference between the two groups, other than the presence of cataracts, was that the cataract-free individuals had taken at least 400 international units (one regular capsule) of vitamin E and/or a minimum of 300 milligrams of vitamin C per day over the last five years," the report says.

Most of the cataract-free people took only one of the two vitamins in the form of supplements. Those who took extra vitamin C showed a risk reduction of 70 percent, the report says. Those who took vitamin E supplements had a 50 percent reduction in cataract risk.

This study backs up other recent research that also shows dramatic blindness prevention benefits for people using these two vitamins. One doctor, Charles Kelman, recommends taking 1,000 to 2,000 milligrams (one to two grams) of vitamin C (ascorbic acid) daily to help prevent cataracts. Scientists don't know for sure why the vitamins prevent cloudy formations in aging eyes. Those clouds across the field of vision are caused by proteins being oxidized in the lens of the eye and then clumping together.

Some researchers believe that vitamins C and E, both of which are antioxidants, neutralize the lens proteins before they can clump together.

Two out of every 10 people between the ages of 60 and 75 in the United States have cataracts. The condition, which can lead to blindness, accounts for a half million surgical operations every year.

"If you could delay cataract formation by just 10 years, you would eliminate the need for half of the cataract extractions," according to Allen Taylor, who works for the USDA Human Nutrition Research Center on Aging in Medford, Mass.

Things that might cause or trigger cataracts include sunlight (ultra-violet rays), diabetes, steroids and X-rays.

However, vitamins C and E aren't the only powerful natural cataract fighters available. Beta-carotene and ribo-flavin (vitamin B2) also might help prevent the eye-clouding growths. People with higher than average intakes of vitamin C, vitamin E and beta-carotene (known as antioxidant vitamins) "are at a reduced risk of cataract development," according to H. Gerster in a German study (Z. *Ernahrungswiss* 28,1:56).

Other studies by P. Jacques confirm that people with "high levels of at least two of the three vitamins (C, E and B2)" are at reduced risk of developing cataracts compared to people with low levels of these vitamins, reports *Archives of Ophthalmology* (106,3:337).

Harold Skalka has found that a deficiency of riboflavin (vitamin B2) can lead to cataract development, especially in older adults. "Older cataract patients had more riboflavin deficiency. An absence of riboflavin deficiency was found in our older patients with clear lenses," Skalka reports in *The American Journal of Clinical Nutrition* (34,5:861).

In earlier studies (*The Lancet*, 8054:12-3), Skalka suggested that cataracts "may be corrected by dietary restrictions or supplements" of riboflavin. However, "large doses of niacin (vitamin B3) may ... increase the chances of getting cataracts," according to *Vitamin Side Effects Revealed* by FC&A Publishing.

This vitamin can help prevent blindness

Your grandmother was right when she told you to eat your carrots because they're good for your eyes.

Yellow vegetables like carrots are high in vitamin A. One early symptom of a vitamin-A deficiency is loss of vision in near darkness.

So to prevent night blindness, regularly eat vegetables high in vitamin A.

Caffeine may complicate eye problems

Coffee drinkers, beware! That third cup of caffeinated

coffee might be affecting your vision.

Researchers at the University of Texas and Emory University found that the caffeine in coffee can increase pressure in your eyes, which can aggravate problems related to glaucoma.

The first two cups of coffee don't seem to bother the eyes. It's the third, fourth and fifth cups that cause problems.

So people with glaucoma-related eye problems should limit their coffee intake to two cups or less each day, the report suggests.

CHAPTER 38

Vitamins, Minerals and You

You can watch your skin for signs of nutritional deficiencies that even your doctor might not see, reports Dr. Kenneth Neldner, chairman of the Dermatology Department at Texas Tech University.

Here are early-warning signs to watch for: scaly skin, canker sores, wounds that heal slowly and cracks in the corners of the mouth.

Researchers are discovering that even minor nutrition problems show up in the skin, sometimes long before a doctor might see the underlying cause, reports an article in the Dec. 4, 1990 *Atlanta Journal*.

Here are some common deficiencies and their skin signs.

Vitamin C shortage—bleeding gums, soreness in mouth and gums, or a rough, scaly rash around hair roots.

Vitamin B complex deficiency—cracks and canker sores in the corners of the mouth.

Psoriasis and eczema—these skin problems might not be caused by nutrient shortages, but sometimes they can be successfully treated by taking fish oil. Fish oil contains fatty acids, which help the body fight inflammation caused by the two skin conditions.

Skin cancers — deficiencies in zinc, copper, selenium and vitamins A and E increase the risks of developing various skin cancers, the report says.

Because five out of six medical schools don't even offer a formal course in nutrition for medical students, many doctors don't recognize early signs of nutrition problems, says Dr. Neldner.

Don't try to medicate yourself.

If you have some of the possible early warning signs, tell your doctor about this nutritional research and ask that she look at your condition more closely.

RDAs for vitamin A

Vitamin A is essential for your health, but if you get too little or too much, it can be very dangerous. The RDA for vitamin A is as follows:

Infants	375 micrograms
Children ages 1–3	400 micrograms
Children ages 4–6	500 micrograms
Children ages 7–10	700 micrograms
Males, ages 11–51+	1,000 micrograms
Females ages 11–51+	800 micrograms
Pregnant females	800 micrograms
Nursing mothers, 1st 6 months	1,300 micrograms
Nursing mothers, 2nd 6 months	1,200 micrograms

The amounts in the preceding chart are micrograms (one-millionth of a gram) of retinol equivalents (RE). Retinol is the dietary form of vitamin A. One RE equals six micrograms of beta-carotene, the previtamin form of vitamin A that the body converts into as much vitamin A as needed.

Eyes give away deficiency

Night blindness or loss of vision in near darkness is the earliest symptom of a vitamin-A deficiency. A severe deficiency of vitamin A might cause xerophthalmia (dry eyes) and can lead to permanent blindness if the eye tissue becomes ulcerated.

Other symptoms of vitamin-A deficiency are dry, brittle hair; cracked, dry or blemished skin; itching or burning eyes; thickened eyelids; increased infections; softening of tooth enamel; loss of sense of smell; cloudy eye whites; and eventually, in extreme cases, disintegration of the eyeball, says *Vitamin Side Effects Revealed*. The lungs, digestive system and the urinary or reproductive systems might also deteriorate.

Increased cases of respiratory disease, severe diarrhea, and measles that can lead to early deaths are also associated with vitamin-A deficiency.

Although vitamin-A deficiency is not as common in North America or Western Europe as in poor countries, recent studies have shown that more than 20 percent of the population in those areas were receiving less than 70 percent of the RDA and could be suffering from deficiency symptoms.

Smoking, drinking alcohol, or long-term intestinal disease also can increase the body's need for vitamin A.

Natural sources of vitamin A or carotene are liver, cod liver oil, eggs, milk and dairy products, broccoli, spinach and other green, leafy vegetables, carrots, turnips and other yellow vegetables, apricots and cantaloupe. Meats naturally contain vitamin A, while plants contain a "previtamin" form that the body manufactures into vitamin A.

Beta carotene is the natural raw ingredient in some foods that the body works on to turn it into full-blown vitamin A. It's a harmless nutrient — known also as previtamin A — that is found in rich supply in many yellow and green vegetables.

The best part is that carotene usually is not converted into vitamin A unless the body really needs more of the vitamin. It's just burned as food energy or passes on through the body. Therefore, you can eat a lot of carotene and not suffer the same bad effect as you would from eating a lot of vitamin A. But your body normally would still get all the benefits of vitamin A without the dangers.

Also, a recent study in the *Journal of Food Science* (52,4: 1022) has shown that "the carotene content of wet vegetables, either fresh or cooked, was always significantly greater than that of dried ones."

Overdoses of vitamin A can be caused by eating too much animal liver over a period of several weeks. Typically, eating too much animal liver can cause long-lasting headaches and blurring of vision. But usually overdoses are the results of high doses of vitamin supplements, Bendich and Langseth report in *The American Journal of Clinical Nutrition* (49,2:358) — in other words, taking too many vitamin pills.

Vitamin A in the form of pills and supplements can cause more damage to the body than vitamin A and carotene consumed directly from regular food sources. That's because "dietary vitamin A is ingested throughout the day at meals, whereas supplemental vitamin A is usually taken as a single dose of preformed vitamin A in a multivitamin," the study says.

A new study from the Human Nutrition Research Center on Aging shows that "elderly people who take vitamin A supplements might be at increased risk for vitamin A overload." Adults taking repeated daily doses of around ten times the RDA have reported harmful side effects like buildup of pressure within the skull, vomiting, irritability, peeling of skin, loss of hair, dry skin and cracked lips, reports *Vitamin Side Effects Revealed* (FC&A Publishing). Megadoses can cause a toxic reaction or even, in rare cases, death.

Infants given large doses of vitamin A might suffer from itching, dehydration, muscle tremors, soft spots in the skull, and poor heart rhythm from high levels of blood calcium associated with vitamin A poisoning.

Vitamin A is fat-soluble. That means it dissolves in body fat. Because of that, it can be stored in the body for a long time, unlike water-soluble vitamins that are quickly flushed out of the body by the kidneys. The liver can store several months' supply of vitamin A (about 200,000 I.U.), so the amount of vitamin A in the body can become extremely high over many years, researchers at Tufts University report in *The American Journal of Clinical Nutrition* (49,1:112).

"Our study suggests that elderly people should limit their intake of supplemental vitamin A, particularly over the long term," warns Stephen Krasinski, who headed the research team. "Our data might also indirectly support a lowering of the RDA for vitamin A."

The good news about vitamin A overdose is that most bad symptoms will go away when the high doses are stopped. In some cases permanent damage does occur, but usually if the overdose can be diagnosed, and the additional vitamin A eliminated, the recovery will be quite rapid.

Here are some ways to avoid vitamin A overdoses:

- If you take a vitamin supplement, check the fine print on the bottle. Be sure that you never take more than the RDA for vitamin A unless your doctor specifically says it's okay.
- Do not take vitamin A supplements if you are taking cod liver oil or fish oil supplements. Both contain high levels of vitamin A. Cod liver oil or other fish oil should be used with caution, and under your doctor's supervision, because of the risk of vitamin A overdose.
- Do not take more than the RDA of vitamin A if you are elderly, unless your doctor recommends larger doses to correct a deficiency.
- If you want to supplement your body's store of vitamin A, take carotene supplements instead of vitamin A supplements.
- Do not take vitamin A supplements if you are

taking isotretinoin (brand name Accutane) or etretinate (brand name Tegison). Both are prescription drugs that are made from vitamin A.

- Do not take vitamin A supplements if you are on birth control pills, unless you also are under a doctor's supervision. Women taking birth control pills usually show an increase in levels of vitamin A in their blood of 30 to 80 percent, says *Vitamin Side Effects Revealed*.

- Remember to always report your vitamin and mineral supplements to your doctor and, in the case of a medical emergency, the hospital staff.

An internal insect repellant?

Taking vitamin-B1 supplements, known as thiamine, might provide a natural repellant against insects.

In a small study at Michigan's Lake Superior State College, thiamine supplements seemed to protect volunteers from mosquito bites.

Students took the supplement or a placebo (a fake supplement) immediately before they went out into the woods and then kept track of the number of mosquito bites they received.

There were fewer mosquito bites on people who took the thiamine, and now researchers are trying to duplicate the study with more people, to confirm the results.

Niacin safeguards

High-dose niacin, in whatever form it's taken, is a drug, not a vitamin anymore, warns Denise Arthurs of the Tufts University Nutrition Center in Boston.

"At the levels recommended by popular [nutrition] books and by people in the lay public—1,500 [or] 2,000 [or] 3,000 milligrams — niacin ceases to be a vitamin and is, in fact, a drug," Arthurs says. "It has side effects, like most drugs do."

She urged that such high doses be taken only under the direction and constant monitoring of a doctor, reports *Medical Tribune* (31,16:14).

Niacin in high doses should be avoided by some diabetics, warns a report in the *Journal of the American Medical Association* (264,6:723).

Megadose niacin does dramatically lower cholesterol levels, including LDL ("bad") cholesterol.

But, people with non-insulin-dependent diabetes might suffer from a niacin side-effect, the report says.

Niacin treatment in this form of diabetes causes a loss of control of blood sugar levels.

The researchers recommended caution in using nicotinic acid for these diabetics.

Folic acid safety levels

Daily 5- to 15-milligram supplements of folic acid appear safe for healthy people, according to a report in *The*

American Journal of Clinical Nutrition (50,2:353).

Folic acid, one of eight vitamins in the vitamin B complex, is vital to red-blood-cell production. It is found in medications used to treat everything from psoriasis to AIDS.

Scientists say more studies are needed to determine whether folic acid supplements cause toxicity in these patients or decrease a medication's effectiveness.

Folic acid overdose might mask symptoms of severe anemia and interfere with zinc absorption. Pregnant women taking supplements should be sure to get enough zinc as well.

The official RDA for folic acid is 200 micrograms for men and 180 micrograms for women.

B6 allowances

If you are over 50, you might be short-changing yourself on vitamin B6, suggests a report in *The American Journal of Clinical Nutrition* (50,2:391).

Recommended daily allowances (RDAs) of vitamins and minerals are based on the needs of young, healthy adults, say Danish researchers.

The current RDA for B6 is 2.2 milligrams for men and 2.0 milligrams for women.

The researchers suggest that RDAs for the elderly be based on the older person's individual needs.

Those needs likely are different from those of a young person.

The scientists are concerned specifically about vitamin B6, the levels of which decrease in the body with increasing age, sometimes leading to a deficiency.

Vitamin B6 promotes healthy skin, red blood cells and teeth and gums.

Researchers encourage older people to eat more fruits, vegetables and potatoes.

A carefully balanced, healthful diet usually ensures the right amount of B6 and other vitamins.

But people who don't get enough nutrition from their regular diets might need vitamin B6 supplements, the report says.

Women's two vitamin deficiencies masquerade as deadly leukemia

Under the doctor's microscope, the abnormal blood cells seemed to shout one dreaded diagnosis—cancer of the blood, leukemia!

But in two cases, looks were deceiving, even to trained scientists, reports the *British Medical Journal* (300,6734:1263).

After a bone biopsy in one case showed additional leukemia-like cells, doctors at Hammersmith Hospital in London even ordered an intravenous (IV) needle inserted to start chemotherapy.

The 43-year-old woman escaped unnecessary medication when late-arriving blood tests showed she had a severe shortage of vitamin B12 (also known as cobalamin).

That shortage apparently caused pernicious anemia (a lack of nutrient-carrying red blood cells), which also was successfully treated with shots of extra vitamin B12.

Another woman, 52, likewise had abnormal blood and bone-marrow cells, similar to leukemia.

It turned out that she had a shortage of another B-complex vitamin, folate (known to a few people as vitamin B9; another form is folic acid or folacin).

Her anemia also was cured by taking extra folate.

In both cases, after the women got the needed vitamins, their blood tests returned to normal, and the leukemia-like cells disappeared.

Both women had lung or airway infections when they took the blood tests. Doctors speculate that the combination of respiratory infection and anemia might have affected the test results.

Such cases might not happen often, but they do point out the need for extra care in making medical judgments.

The Recommended Dietary Allowance for folate (folacin) is 200 micrograms for men over 51, and 180 micrograms daily for women past age 51.

Natural sources of folate include dark-green, leafy vegetables; liver; dry beans, peanuts; wheat germ and whole grains.

According to the National Research Council publication Diet and Health (1989; pg.67), women tend to take in less folacin daily than men do.

Heat destroys the vitamin, and folate losses caused by cooking and canning can be very high, the report says.

Vitamin B12 comes naturally only in foods of animal origin. Supplying B12 are liver, muscle meats, fish, eggs, milk and milk products.

The RDA for vitamin B12 is two micrograms for men and women over age 51.

Check with your doctor before taking either vitamin B12 or folate supplements.

More good news about 'C'

■ A new role for vitamin C might be in fighting cholesterol-plaque build-up in arteries, suggests a study reported in the *Medical Tribune* (31,16:14).

Vitamin C stays on the job far longer than vitamin E in fighting oxidation of low-density lipoprotein (the "bad" LDL form of cholesterol).

University of Texas researchers believe oxidized LDL triggers atherosclerosis, or hardening of the arteries.

Because vitamin C does such a good job of battling this cholesterol, Dr. Ishwarlal Jialal suggests that the RDA should be doubled, from 60 milligrams to 120, the article says.

Hardening of the arteries causes heart disease and some strokes.

■ Vitamin C's best-known prevention role probably is its ability to neutralize several cancer-causing chemicals in cooked and processed foods.

It also acts as an antioxidant against so-called free radicals. Free radicals are tissue-harming substances brought into the bloodstream by food, air pollution and tobacco smoke.

More 'C' needed?

Your arteries might need more vitamin C than current government guidelines call for, according to a report in *Science News* (136,9:133).

Scientists at the University of California at Berkeley are calling for an increase in the recommended daily allowance of vitamin C, after studies there showed that vitamin C neutralizes toxic chemicals in the blood that initiate hardening of the arteries.

"I was quite surprised at how much better a scavenger of free radicals [vitamin C] was, especially when compared to vitamin E," says biochemist Balz Frei.

Vitamin C performed even better than naturally occurring substances in the blood that fight toxic intruders, the report says.

Vitamin D needs increase with age

Elderly Americans, especially those who are bedridden, might need higher amounts of vitamin D to prevent rickets-like disease, according to a report in *Drug Therapy* (19,8:63).

Studies suggest that with increasing age, the skin cannot produce vitamin D efficiently. In addition, the intestines cannot effectively absorb supplements, the report says.

Sun exposure increases vitamin D production in the body, but in one study, even people living in sunny climates had lower vitamin D levels.

Vegetarians need vitamins

People on strict vegetarian diets might run a greater risk of developing vitamin B12 and vitamin D deficiencies than non-vegetarians.

According to a report in *The American Journal of Clinical Nutrition* (50,4:718), a recent French study indicates that vegetarians and non-vegetarians had equal amounts of thiamin, riboflavin, folates and vitamins B6, A, and E.

However, the vegetarians had lower amounts of vitamin B12 and vitamin D than the non-vegetarians.

To prevent vitamin deficiencies, vegetarians should eat more vitamin B-12 and vitamin D rich foods or consider taking vitamin supplements to complement their diet.

The goods on vitamin E

Sources: Green leafy vegetables, shrimp and other seafood, margarine, nuts, vegetable oils, apples, apricots, peaches, wheat germ and whole-wheat flour.

Function: Promotes normal growth and development; helps reduce tissue damage after exercise; helps prevent atherosclerosis; acts as an anti-clotting agent in the blood; helps protect blood cells from oxidation (cell damage).

Who needs more of it: People over the age of 55; those who exercise regularly; people with hyperthyroidism; those with alcohol or other drug abuse.

Deficiency: Anemia, inability to concentrate, muscle weakness or damage, irritability, lack of energy and vitality, decreased sexual performance.

Too much: Possible increase in level of cholesterol in the blood; increased chance of blood clots; impairs sexual function; changes immune system responses, higher death rates.

Recommended daily allowance: Men over age 50 need 10 milligrams daily; women over age 50 need 8 milligrams daily.

Source: *FDA Consumer* (24,9:31)

Vitamin E and smoking

Worried about secondary smoke in the workplace or at home?

A study reported in *Alive* (Feb/March 1990:1) suggests that taking more vitamin E might reduce chances of lung damage.

Cigarette smoke creates free radicals, which are tiny particles that can cause lung tissue damage.

The free radicals make it difficult for your lungs to turn the air you breathe into usable oxygen for the blood system. Free radical damage has been linked directly to the development of lung cancer, emphysema and chronic bronchitis.

Vitamin E helps trap these free radicals and prevents

them from harming the delicate lung tissue.

So, if you can't escape smoke from other people's cigarettes, vitamin E might be your best defense against lung disease.

Be sure to check with your doctor before you start taking extra vitamin E.

Exercisers need more 'E'

If you exercise regularly, you probably need to eat more green, leafy vegetables, and more apples and apricots.

These foods contain large amounts of vitamin E, and studies suggest that people who exercise regularly need more vitamin E than those who do not exercise with any regularity, reports *Nutrition Today* (25,5 :5).

Due to the muscular stress that accompanies many types of exercise, most people experience slight muscle damage during exercise.

Based on recent studies, researchers report that vitamin E helps minimize tissue damage that could be caused by exercise and then helps restore muscles to a healthy state after exercise.

If you exercise regularly, talk to your doctor about your daily intake of vitamin E. He can advise you on how much vitamin E you should be taking in daily to minimize muscular damage and maximize the benefits of your exercise.

Calcium for your bones

As odd as it might sound, perfectly healthy women in their 30s could be losing calcium out of their bones. In later life, this could lead to a stooped posture and easily broken bones.

This does not sound too serious until you realize that as many as 50,000 people a year die from complications associated with osteoporosis, the name given to the chronic loss of calcium from the bones.

Many experts now recommend that women consume at least 1,000 milligrams (one gram) of calcium per day. Children and pregnant women should increase that figure to 1,200 milligrams.

That is equivalent to drinking about three and one-third cups of low-fat milk a day for most women, and four cups of milk per day for pregnant women.

Milk is by no means the only way to consume calcium. Any dairy product, including cottage cheese and yogurt, will work. Cheese is a good choice if you select low-fat varieties. Adding dry milk to bread recipes and using a baking mix that contains dry milk are other choices.

Non-dairy products, including beans, tofu, lentils and several of the greens (mustard and collards), are also excellent sources.

Calcium has other benefits as well

■ Heart disease. In one study, women who took 800

milligrams of calcium every day decreased their high blood pressure by 23 percent.

Women taking only 400 milligrams did not benefit as much.

High blood pressure is a serious heart-disease risk factor.

■ Bone disease. It's no secret that calcium promotes strong teeth and bones — but not just when you're young.

Dr. Robert P. Heany, of Creighton University in Omaha, Nebraska, notes the importance of calcium in two major stages of life:

(1) It helps develop bone mass during the first 30 years of life, and

(2) then maintains bone mass during the remaining years of life.

However, as you get older, your body doesn't use calcium as efficiently as when you were young.

That's why you might need more calcium as you age, some researchers suggest.

Menopausal women might need even more calcium because their estrogen loss puts them at greater risk of developing osteoporosis.

■ For pregnant women, extra calcium might help prevent preeclampsia. This condition results in excessive fluid retention in the mother's body, which can kill the unborn child if not treated.

Have your calcium supplements passed the vinegar test?

If not, your body might not be getting the benefit of what you're feeding it, suggests a report in *Nutrition Action Health Letter* (17,5:1).

The vinegar test can show how quickly and completely your calcium tablet crumbles and dissolves.

If your tablet flunks the test in vinegar, it probably won't dissolve in your body either, says the report.

Here's how to find out whether you're getting the nutrients you're paying for:

Put one tablet in a glass of plain apple-cider vinegar. That's to simulate the acid environment of your stomach, the first stop for anything you take by mouth.

Time how long it takes the tablet to completely disintegrate (crumble apart).

In addition, measure how long it takes for the crumbled tablet to dissolve in the liquid and become part of the liquid solution.

Crumbling time of an hour or more might indicate a problem.

If the tablet hasn't crumbled by the time it leaves your stomach, the calcium carbonate likely won't get absorbed into your bloodstream, says the *Nutrition Action* report.

Dissolving time of more than a half-day should be a warning sign, whether regular or timed-release forms of calcium.

Try a similar test with your other vitamin-mineral supplements.

Drop a tablet into just a glass of plain water.

Again, if it takes more than four or five hours to dissolve, much, if not most, of the nutrients will just pass on through your system without getting absorbed.

"Tablets that do disintegrate may not get into the bloodstream," the reports quotes University of Maryland researcher Ralph Shangraw. "But if it doesn't disintegrate, that's a pretty good indication that it won't get absorbed."

Shangraw calls for much quicker crumbling times — under 30 minutes.

Some brands do better than others.

Supplements with potentially poor dissolving rates include generic-brand multi-vitamins and multi-minerals, timed- or slow-release tablets and big, solid pills like calcium-magnesium-zinc combinations.

Some slow-release tablets might not dissolve at all.

The report tells of one supplement user who opened his septic tank for repair and discovered a layer of undissolved vitamin pills.

Generally, capsules out-perform solid tablets or pills, usually because capsules have a gelatin outer-skin that dissolves quickly in the stomach.

Liquid forms, of course, are the most quickly absorbed.

Manganese
Needed: more of that other 'M' mineral

Most of us need more of another "trace" mineral: manganese. It's an important fighter against osteoporosis (dangerous bone loss among older persons, especially women over 50). It also acts like a traffic cop to insulin, signaling how much to produce and when to release it into the bloodstream, and helps heal tissue damage caused by ozone and other environmental pollutants.

Studies reported in *Science News* (130:199) indicate the body has trouble absorbing manganese even when we eat enough of the right foods. Further, even the recommended dietary allowance (RDA) of 2.0 to 5.0 milligrams per day might be too low. A University of Texas research project involving tests on people showed that one must eat at least 3.8 milligrams each day to keep from running low on the mineral.

The problem is that other ingredients in manganese-rich foods — like spinach, wheat bran, and tea — cause the mineral to slip through the digestive tract without much of it being absorbed. The manganese present in meats, milk, and eggs, though in smaller amounts than in other foods, is more easily absorbed, which makes these "bio-available" sources of the mineral more important in a nutritious diet.

A better approach might be to take manganese supplements in the form of daily tablets, but watch when you take it and with what other minerals. Studies show that mineral supplements containing iron, calcium, and magnesium cut down on the body's absorption of manganese. So if you take manganese, for best effect, wait several hours before taking other kinds of mineral tablets.

The tip-off to the link between bone problems and manganese deficiency occurred to biologist Paul Saltman after he studied the chronic bone fractures suffered by basketball superstar Bill Walton. X-rays showed Walton had a form of osteoporosis, resulting in continuous bone loss and breakage. Blood tests showed the athlete had no manganese and half the normal levels of zinc and copper. The researcher took Walton off his macrobiotic diet and put him on mineral supplements, and within six weeks Walton resumed his career playing basketball.

The mineral plays an important role in helping specialized cells break down old bone tissue and replace it with new bone cells. A manganese deficiency weakens the bone-building cells, resulting in increasingly porous bones and symptoms of osteoporosis, the report said. Another study of Belgium women with severe osteoporosis showed the women had one-fourth the manganese levels in their blood as women of the same age without the bone disease.

The moral of the story is clear: supplement your diet with manganese-rich foods, and be careful not to take it with blocking agents like magnesium, iron, calcium, phytate and fiber in bran, oxalic acid in things like spinach, and tannins in tea.

Selenium

Men seem to be more sensitive to a deficiency of the mineral nutrient selenium.

Men with lower levels of selenium in their blood were more likely to develop cancers of the lung, stomach and pancreas, reports the *Journal of the National Cancer Institute* (82,10:864).

That finding comes from a big, 10-year Finnish study of nearly 40,000 men and women.

Women had a marginally higher risk because of low selenium, but not nearly so much as men, according to researcher Paul Knekt.

Men who averaged 59.1 micrograms of selenium per liter of blood had the highest risk. Men with an average of 62.5 micrograms had the lowest risk, the report says.

People in Finland, a Scandinavian country bordering the former Soviet Union, don't get much selenium in their diets, the report says.

The U.S. Recommended Dietary Allowance (RDA) for selenium is 70 micrograms daily for men over 50, and 55 micrograms for women 51 and above.

More selenium snapshots

■ Low selenium levels also seem to be linked in some way to bladder cancer.

Thirty-five people developed bladder cancer out of a group of 25,802 people that researchers were keeping tabs on.

Those with bladder cancer had significantly lower blood levels of selenium than people who were cancer-free, according to a digest of a study in *Cancer Research* (49,21:6144).

■ In another Scandinavian country, Sweden, researchers measured blood levels of selenium in people who were being treated for diseases of the heart and digestive system.

The biggest shortages were found among those with

digestive diseases, according to a digest of a report in the *Journal of Internal Medicine* (225:85).

People with stomach and intestinal diseases might have selenium deficiency, the report indicates. A selenium shortage could further harm their immune systems and delay their recovery.

They might need selenium supplements, the report suggests.

■ Two studies suggest that low selenium levels might contribute to the development of asthma or even partly cause it.

People with symptoms of asthma have lower levels of selenium in their blood and blood plasma, says a British study reported in *Clinical Science* (77,5:495).

In New Zealand, people with the lowest levels of selenium are twice as likely to develop asthma as those with the highest levels.

Also, those with low levels of glutathione peroxidase had five times the asthma risk, says a study in the British scientific journal *Thorax* (45:95).

Glutathione peroxidase is a natural, anti-inflammatory enzyme produced by the body.

Selenium forms part of the chemical makeup of this enzyme, which battles the inflammation of lung tissues caused by asthma.

A New Zealander typically gets less than 30 micrograms a day of selenium.

■ Selenium apparently works closely with vitamin E, a powerful antioxidant, to neutralize harmful free radicals circulating in the blood.

Natural sources of selenium include Brazil nuts, salmon, tuna, swordfish, shrimp, lobster, oysters, whole grains and sunflower seeds.

Brazil nuts are an especially rich source, mainly because they are grown in soil high in selenium.

In fact, a quarter-ounce of Brazil nut meat — about the size of one nut — provides 76.8 micrograms of selenium, well above the RDA.

But, be aware that one Brazil nut is about 85 percent fat, one-third of that saturated fat.

Check with your doctor before taking a selenium supplement.

Even small amounts above the RDA can cause side effects like nail damage, hair loss, nausea, diarrhea, skin odor, fatigue, irritability and even damage to the nervous system, says *Recommended Dietary Allowances, 10th Edition* (National Research Council, 1989:pg.221).

Sodium in your diet

While you are increasing calcium consumption, you might be among those who have been told to reduce the amount of sodium in the diet.

Everyone needs some sodium because it aids the body in absorbing nutrients. It also plays a major role in maintaining normal blood volume.

But if you have high blood pressure (hypertension), and your doctor has told you to restrict your sodium intake, you should find ways to limit it.

When reading any recipe, be on the lookout for salt, canned products, many of the condiments and other items that are high in sodium.

Keep in mind that salt is not just sodium. Common table salt is sodium chloride and contains about 40 percent sodium.

On a can label, many different sodiums such as sodium saccharin or sodium hydroxide might be listed. These ingredients should be avoided as well.

Other tell-tale ingredients to avoid include soda, baking soda and MSG (monosodium glutamate).

Zinc: good and bad

Low levels of zinc can reduce your body's immune response and increase your risk of infections. A zinc deficiency can even cause you to lose excessive amounts of hair.

But too much zinc can reduce the effectiveness of copper, iron and other minerals in your system.

A study in *Journal of Nutrition for the Elderly* (8,1:3) indicates that the RDA (or recommended dietary allowance) provides enough zinc to keep a normal person's immune system responding well without harming the needed absorption of other minerals.

Adult men over 50 should get 15 milligrams of zinc daily, while women should get 12 milligrams, the RDA according to the federal government. Liver, seafood (especially herring and shellfish), dairy products, meat, whole grains and eggs are good sources of zinc, while vegetables are poor sources of zinc.

Adequate zinc consumption might actually help to lower death rates. That's because a less healthy immune system results in more infections among elderly people. And more infections result in higher death rates for seniors.

Zinc also might help prevent "macular degeneration," a deterioration of the nerves in the eyes. In a study at the Louisiana State University Eye Center, older adults who took zinc supplements for up to two years had less eye deterioration than people who didn't receive the supplements.

In addition, zinc also has been reported to help fight cancer and skin disease, to improve the sense of taste, and to shorten the length of the common cold, says the *Journal of Nutrition for the Elderly* (8,2:49).

If you experience an unexplained loss of hair, you might want to check for a zinc deficiency. Eating more meats, especially organ meats like calves' liver, could solve the problem.

Aging alone does not cause low levels of zinc, according to *The American Journal of Clinical Nutrition* (48,2:343).

Since many elderly people reduce their food intake, researchers believe that older people, especially those in institutions, are not usually getting the minimum daily requirement for zinc.

A study at Bowling Green State University found that "dietary zinc intakes were inadequate in 67 percent" of the elderly.

The journal *Human Nutrition and Applied Nutrition* (40,6:440) reports that in one acute medical care ward studied, the meals served by the institution provided only about one-half the RDA of zinc — even if the patient ate everything on the plate!

Phytic acid, found in grains and other dietary fiber, interferes with the absorption of zinc, so people on high fiber or vegetarian diets might not get adequate amounts of zinc. Normal cooking "decreases the phytic acid content and improves zinc absorption," says *The Journal of Nutrition* (117,11:1898).

Zinc supplements above the RDA interfere with the body's metabolism of copper and iron.

"Many women might be at risk for iron deficiency" even with supplements of less than four times the RDA of zinc, says *The American Journal of Clinical Nutrition* (49,1:145).

Decreased levels of copper, which helps in the formation of bone, hair and skin and is important in the formation of hemoglobin and red blood cells, are also caused by excessive doses of zinc supplements.

While the proper amount of zinc greatly helps the body's immune system, too much zinc has the opposite effect. Excessive intake of zinc is suspected to impair the immune system's response, says the *Journal of the American Medical Association* (252,11:1443).

Too much zinc also lowers the level of "good" cholesterol known as HDL, according to *Metabolism* (34:519).

Consuming the RDA of zinc is essential for good health. But high doses should be avoided because of its effects on other minerals and because of possible negative effects on cholesterol levels and the immune system.

CHAPTER 39

Weight Loss

Obesity: How much weight are you making your body carry?

Blood pressure levels increase in proportion to the number of pounds someone is overweight, according to researchers who studied the residents of Framingham, Massachusetts, for more than 10 years. It is more difficult for the heart to pump the blood in an overweight person because the heart must pump more blood through more tissue.

But how heavy is too heavy? Most medical professionals describe obesity as being 20 to 40 percent heavier than your ideal weight. However, health professionals warn that if you are 10 pounds over your ideal weight, you are overweight. About one-fourth of the U.S. population is more than 20 percent over desired weight, according to the Centers for Disease Control in Atlanta.

Since the heavier you are, the higher your risk of developing high blood pressure, obesity is one of the major causes of high blood pressure. However, the Framingham study also found that blood pressure dropped significantly when weight was lost. So just by gaining or losing weight, you can affect your blood pressure.

Remember that measuring pounds and ounces is not the only way to determine who is fat. Body builders, athletes and people who do hard manual labor are often heavier than their "ideal" weight, but they are not overweight. Since muscle weighs more than fat, you can be heavier without being fat. If you can "pinch an inch" you need to lose weight. The pinch test can be used on the underneath of your upper arm or on your stomach. However, usually the pinch test is not necessary because most people know when they are overweight. The hard part is just admitting it to ourselves and doing something about it.

People with mild high blood pressure who lost just 10 pounds were able to stop taking medicine to control their blood pressure in a recent study, according to *Better Health* (5,8). A different research team found a direct relationship with the amount of weight lost and the reduction in blood pressure. They found that with every seven pounds lost, the top number (systolic blood pressure level) will drop seven points and the bottom number (diastolic) will drop four points.

What is your ideal weight?

It is determined by your age, height and sex. The weight chart that follows is based on the life-expectancy by sex at certain ages, weights and heights. They show that "ideal" weights increase as we get older. Note that there is no such thing as one "ideal" weight for any height or age. Rather, normal weights fall within a "range" that can vary 40 pounds or more.

Height Feet and Inches	Acceptable Weight (in pounds)			
	35 Yr	45 Yr	55 Yr	65 Yr
4 10	92-119	99-127	107-135	115-142
4 11	95-123	103-131	111-139	119-147
5 0	98-127	106-135	114-143	123-152
5 1	101-131	110-140	118-148	127-157
5 2	105-136	113-144	122-153	131-163
5 3	108-140	117-149	126-158	135-168
5 4	112-145	121-154	130-163	140-173
5 5	115-149	125-159	134-168	144-179
5 6	119-154	129-164	138-174	148-184
5 7	122-159	133-169	143-179	153-190
5 8	126-163	137-174	147-184	158-196
5 9	130-168	141-179	151-190	162-201
5 10	134-173	145-184	156-195	167-207
5 11	137-178	149-190	160-201	172-213
6 0	141-183	153-195	165-207	177-219
6 1	145-188	157-200	169-213	182-225
6 2	149-194	162-206	174-219	187-232
6 3	153-199	166-212	179-225	192-238
6 4	157-205	171-218	184-231	197-244

*Table values are for height without shoes and weight without clothes.

Source: Baltimore Longitudinal Study of Aging, conducted at the Gerontology Research Center, National Institute on Aging.

Here are some tips on how to change your eating habits so you can maintain a healthy weight:

• Avoid crash diets and dangerous weight-loss schemes. Choose a diet that you can live with for the rest of your life. Once someone goes off a severe diet, they usually binge to meet all their cravings that have not been fulfilled. Cycles of rapid weight loss, weight gain, weight loss and weight gain are extremely hard on the body's organs, can lead to high blood pressure, and can be dangerous to your overall health. Gradual weight loss that can be maintained is the healthiest way to lose weight.

• Keep a food journal of what, how much and when you eat each day. With a journal you can see exactly where your calories and nutrition are coming from and how you can alter your eating habits.

• Weigh yourself once a week and record it in your food journal. Daily fluctuations in weight are not reliable, but a weekly weighing will allow you to evaluate if your program is working.

• Set a realistic goal weight for yourself, preferably with your doctor's endorsement. Being overweight is dangerous, but so is being underweight. Each person has a different metabolism that burns calories at slightly different rates. Choose a weight that is safe and healthy for your height, age and lifestyle.

• Choose specific times to eat your meals and snacks, and do not eat at any other time. Never skip meals because you will be inclined to eat more at the next meal to make up the difference.

• Do not eat if you are not hungry. As children, we were

often required to eat "everything on our plates" and ate even when we were not hungry, but these patterns can lead to obesity.

- Learn to say "no" without feeling guilty. Once again, do not let someone coerce you into eating.

- Eat slowly. Put your utensils down after each bite. It takes several minutes for the stomach to tell the brain that it is full, so eating slowly will help you to realize you're full before you overeat.

- Try to reduce your intake of all food rather than completely restricting yourself to certain foods. If you are not allowed to have a specific item, usually you will crave that "forbidden fruit." This is particularly true when working with overweight children. It is best to learn good overall eating habits rather than prohibiting certain foods for the rest of their lives.

- Drink grapefruit juice, unsalted (a low-sodium brand) tomato juice or unsweetened lemonade as an appetizer before your meal. If you allow 20 minutes before you eat, the acid in the juice will help you feel full, and you will be able to eat less. Drink the juice of a whole lemon squeezed into a glass of water, twice a day, for another natural appetite suppressant.

- Serve your meals on smaller plates so they will look fuller.

- Put the food on the plates away from the table. If you bring serving dishes to the table, you will be more tempted to have additional helpings.

- Avoid dishes and table settings that are bright because bright colors may stimulate the appetite.

- Never eat food out of the original container. Take out an

appropriate serving and return the container to its proper place. By eating directly out of the container, you are more likely to eat too much.

- Try to leave something on your plate. In some oriental countries this is considered a high compliment because it shows that you have had plenty to eat. If you have been raised to clear your plate and not to "waste food," learning to leave a small portion on your plate will be good for you.

- Switch to lower calorie foods like skim milk and calorie-reduced products.

- Many doctors now recommend avoiding products with artificial sweeteners. Although they seem to be a boon for dieters, some doctors believe that artificial sweeteners increase or maintain the desire for sweets which is not helpful to someone who is dieting.

  Using artificial sweeteners does not guarantee weight loss, reports new research by the American Cancer Society. In a study of 78,000 dieters, people using artificial sweeteners gained more weight than people not using substitutes. The artificial sweeteners did not cause the weight gain. However, the researchers concluded that the people thought they were cutting back by using the artificial sweeteners, and they just didn't limit their calories overall. Don't be lulled into a false sense of security — reducing total caloric intake and exercising are the only true ways to lose weight.

- Avoid diet pills, even prescription drugs, unless your doctor believes they are absolutely necessary. For example, a 37-year-old woman nearly died when her heart stopped, Dr. Harry R. Gibbs reports in *The New England*

Journal of Medicine (318: 17, 1127). The woman had been taking three drugs prescribed for weight loss — phentermine hydrochloride, thyroid, and trichlormethiazide — and didn't have any heart or artery problems. Gibbs warns that using inappropriate prescription drugs to treat obesity, even in someone without heart problems, can lead to "sudden catastrophic events."

- Do not use over-the-counter appetite suppressants. One common ingredient, phenylpropanolamine hydrochloride (PPA), has been found to cause high blood pressure even at the doses recommended for weight loss. Anyone with diabetes, heart disease, thyroid disease or high blood pressure should avoid products containing PPA, recommends the *Health Letter* (2:1).
- Do not use or purchase a product that promises to reduce or remove fat in one specific body area. Except for specific exercise or cosmetic surgery, one part of your body cannot be reduced.
- Do not use a "body wrap" in hopes of losing weight. The only weight loss that body wraps provide is the loss of sweat, which is just temporary. Using body wraps can be harmful because the body's temperature is allowed to escalate, producing the bad effects of a heat stroke.
- Eat more vegetables and smaller portions of meat, especially if it's red meat.
- Trim all noticeable fat from meat, and remove the skin before eating.
- Eat plenty of high-fiber foods like whole-grain products, beans and vegetables.
- Use a low-calorie, soft-spread alternative to butter. If you

use a soft-spread, you'll use less because it spreads easier than butter or margarine.

- Eliminate alcohol because it is high in "empty" calories. Alcohol products contain a lot of calories, but they have no nutritional value. Alcohol consumption is also a contributing factor in high blood pressure.
- Keep healthful snacks available. Try cutting up celery, carrots, broccoli, cauliflower, radishes and whatever other vegetables you like and leaving them in the refrigerator. Buy plenty of fruit. It provides quick and easy snacks.
- Buy high-quality popcorn that tastes good without butter or salt. To flavor your popcorn, try lightly spraying the popcorn with a low-calorie vegetable oil, then add cinnamon, curry powder, onion powder, chili powder or other herbs.
- Reduce or eliminate high-calorie nuts and nut products, including peanut butter.
- Never go grocery shopping when you are hungry. If you are hungry, you will tend to buy more, and you are more easily tempted to buy high-calorie foods.
- Make a shopping list of things you need and stick to it. Don't be seduced by unnecessary foods.
- Don't keep high-calorie foods in your home.
- Don't store food within sight.
- Eat early in the day to achieve your maximum weight loss. Researchers at Tulane Unversity found that people who ate their last meal at least eight hours before they went to sleep lost between five and 10 pounds a month (*Postgraduate Medicine*, 79:4,352). The participants did not change the amount of food they ate, or the number of calories, just

the time of day it was eaten. If you eat most of your daily calories in the morning and at noon, and have a light snack for the evening meal, you should be able to boost your weight loss.

- The Good Wellness Program for Weight Management suggests placing a bottle of mouthwash in front of the refrigerator door. If you stray into the kitchen looking for "something to eat," you will have to move the mouthwash first. The director of the program, suggests rinsing with the mouthwash to satisfy the cravings without consuming any calories.
- Brushing your teeth frequently may help reduce snacking. Your teeth and mouth feel so good that you don't have the desire to eat.
- Remember your diet when eating outside of your home, at a restaurant, or someone else's home. If you eat at a cafeteria, like a school lunchroom, check with the food services manager to see if low-calorie meals can be ordered.
- If you must have dessert, try sharing it with one or two other people. After a fine meal, you do not need the dessert, but a small sample may meet your craving for a sweet.
- When flying or traveling by train, request a low-calorie meal at least 24 hours in advance of your departure.
- Do not reward yourself with food or use food to fight stress or depression. Buy yourself a gift or treat yourself to a favorite activity, rather than using food as a release or reward.
- Try squeezing your earlobe for 60 seconds before eating.

This is a technique of acupressure that may help curb your appetite.

- Obese dieters who lose weight very quickly are at increased risk of developing gallstones, doctors at the Cedars-Sinai Medical Center in Los Angeles report. However, if four aspirins are taken each day, the dieter should not develop gallstones, according to the research. You should discuss the aspirin treatment with your doctor if you are considering a low-calorie diet.

- Exercise alone does not cause weight to "just disappear." However, a regular exercise program will make it easier for you to maintain your weight. Since the most important element of exercising is actually "doing it," it is important that the exercise you choose is something you will continue. According to the Federal Trade Commission, of the people who join a fitness club or health spa, 70 percent will quit within just three months.

Exercise helps some people lose weight because it increases their awareness of their bodies. Many people who start an exercise program are suddenly aware of what and how much they are eating. Exercising (and feeling those tired muscles) can be a good reminder that they are trying to lose weight. If you are faithful to your exercise program, you'll eat better and eat less because you won't want to "undo" the good your exercising has done!

If you decide you need a diet ....

How can you lose weight?

Eat fewer calories and exercise. Most obesity is caused by underexercise rather than overeating, according to a recent report by the U.S. Department of Health and Human Services. The combination of exercise with a proper diet is important to fight obesity. These are very simple rules that can contribute to safe, gradual weight-loss. However, most Americans seem to want a "pill" that they can take so they will be thinner in the morning. Losing weight is a lifelong commitment to proper nutrition and regular exercise. It is not too difficult, although it may be a drastic change from a sedentary lifestyle.

Consult your doctor before starting any weight loss program, especially if you are pregnant, over 60 years old and need to lose 20 pounds or more, or have an immediate family member who has had a heart attack or diabetes.

What in the world are you eating?

Many times when you read about dieting, you are bombarded with information about calories, carbohydrates, fats and protein. What is even more confusing are the different ways these items are combined in different diets.

Sometimes diet books advocate reducing calories without saying which calories to reduce: every day you could conceivably eat a hot fudge sundae and very little else. But what would that do to your health?

In the 1970s, low-carbohydrate diets resurfaced.

"Do not eat many carbohydrates," we were told, "but eat as many eggs and steaks as you wanted."

That was bad advice. A person may lose weight on such a diet, but could end up with arteries plugged full of cholesterol.

Who knows what weird combination will be advocated next, leaving many people just as overweight as ever and even more unhealthy because of an unwise diet?

Recent medical research suggests that you should eat fewer fats and calories, but more complex carbohydrates.

Just what are these carbohydrates, calories and other terms that all the diet people talk about?

Some definitions

• Calorie: scientists would say that one "kilocalorie" is the amount of heat needed to raise the temperature of one kilogram of water one degree centigrade. In popular usage and in this book, however, the technical term "kilocalorie" has been shortened to the more familiar and more popular "calorie."

Thus, we use "calorie" to mean the amount of energy produced by food when utilized by the body. In other words, it is a way to measure the amount of energy that a food will produce in the body.

If a calorie is not used up during normal activity, it is stored in some form in the body for later use. If the amount of calories burned is consistently more than the amount of calories eaten, weight loss will result.

• Carbohydrates: these are energy-producing foods such as sugars, starches and cellulose. Carbohydrates are typically divided into two types.

The first type includes simple and double carbohydrates, such as honey and refined sugars.

The second type consists of complex carbohydrates, such as the starches found in whole grains like oats.

Simple sugars are easily digested and enter the bloodstream rapidly. This may cause difficulty for individuals who have trouble controlling the effects of sugar in the body.

In most people, simple carbohydrates will cause sudden peaking and dropping of blood sugar levels, which could lead to a craving for food and a net loss of energy.

Complex carbohydrates require prolonged action by digestive enzymes before the body can use the energy from these foods. The effects of complex carbohydrates on the body are much more gradual, and are unlikely to lead to drops in blood sugar levels and overeating.

- Fats: for all their bad reputation, fats do play an important role in a healthy body. Also called lipids, fats are the most highly concentrated source of energy in the body. One gram of fat will produce about nine calories for the body's use (or storage).

Fats are also important because they are necessary for the body to utilize vitamins A, D, E and K, as well as calcium. They also protect vital organs and help to insulate the body from changes in the surrounding environment.

As explained in other parts of this guide, too many fats in the diet will lead to excessive weight gain. Such an excess also will slow digestion. And too many saturated fats — the types that are solid at room temperature and usually come from animal sources — may lead to high levels of cholesterol and heart disease.

• Protein: this part of our diet is of vital importance for good health. Protein forms the body's "building blocks" for muscles, blood, skin, internal organs and hair. It is also necessary for both the formation and regulation of hormones.

When proteins are digested, they are broken down into simpler units known as "amino acids." The body can use amino acids only when they appear in certain combinations. These combinations are readily available in most meat and egg products.

The right combination may also be created by combining certain food products. For example, to create a complete protein using a food from the grain family (such as oats), it must be paired with a legume (such as peas).

But too much protein will lead to weight gain. Extra protein in the body can be converted by the liver and stored in body tissues as fat.

Tricks for weight loss

After a little time on a diet, many people find "tricks" that can make dieting seem less difficult. Here are some ideas that many people have found helpful:

• Before beginning your diet, write a list detailing your reasons for following a new eating pattern. Prominent on the list should be the health factors and reasons for wanting to lose (or maintain) weight. Keep the list handy for moments when you want to fall away from the diet.

- Always substitute skim milk for whole milk. Not only is this important for calorie reduction, it also is important for reducing animal fat in your diet. A one-cup serving of whole milk provides 150 calories and 5.07 grams of saturated fat. Skim milk has 86 calories and less than three-tenths of a gram of saturated fat. Both nonfat dry milk and skimmed evaporated milk make good choices when cooking. Both have less than a half-gram of saturated fat.

- Resolve never to consume calories in the things you drink, except for the calories in milk. Water, club soda, decaffeinated tea and coffee are all good no-calorie choices. Most soft drinks and fruit-flavored beverages are loaded with calories and have very little nutrition to offer in return.

- Do not weigh yourself every day. Your weight might fluctuate up for a day without reflecting on the success of your diet. It is more encouraging to weigh yourself only once or twice a week.

- Switch from mayonnaise and egg sauces to nonfat yogurt and low-fat cottage cheese. The yogurt and cottage cheese can produce a creamy base for many sauces with far less fat and calories than mayonnaise.

- Do not skip meals. That leads to poor nutrition. Plus, skipping a meal will leave you hungrier and more likely to overeat later on.

- Make a habit of keeping food out of sight. Do not leave high-calorie snack food in the house. In the refrigerator, place raw vegetables and no-calorie drinks at eye level.

- Before attending receptions and parties, eat a small, very-high-fiber meal. If you are full, you will be less likely to pig-out. Plus, the high-fiber might help reduce your taste for fat-filled foods.

- When you do serve meat, trim away any excess fat. Try grilling or broiling where some of the excess fats drip away during cooking.
- Always, but always, remove skin from chicken and other poultry before cooking. In restaurants, look for menu items that feature chicken fillets that are baked or broiled. Fillets are almost always prepared without skin.
- Do you have favorite places or activities for eating? For example, do you love to consume candy at movie theaters or big, fried-chicken lunches at football games? Try finding new hobbies or take along foods that will not ruin your diet.
- Serve a salad or low-calorie soup with most meals. These will fill you up and make you feel fuller on smaller portions.
- Serve open-faced sandwiches. This will save you the extra calories of a second piece of bread. Always serve whole-grain bread.
- Do not go off the diet or stop exercising just because you do not feel entirely well. However, if you are truly sick, a day off from exercising might be a good idea. And if you have dramatically lowered your daily calorie intake, bring it back up to a less stress-inducing level.
- If you do break your diet, do not let guilt drive you away from your eating regime—even for a day. Read over your reasons for being on the diet in the first place, and pick up again where you left off.

- Never use canned fruit products that have been packaged in heavy syrup. Use fresh fruit or fruit that has been packed in its own, unsweetened juice.
- When eating at a restaurant or social occasion, do not be afraid to leave food on your plate. Simply skip over the foods you know will KO your diet.
- Get out of the habit of watching television while eating meals. Sit down, really enjoy what you are eating, and avoid distractions.

Easy 'OJ diet' might help you lose weight

You don't need to send off for it if you see an ad for an "orange juice diet."

That's because you've got the whole diet right in your supermarket produce section or chilled juice case.

It's simple: scientists have discovered that water mixed with fructose suppresses your appetite better than glucose with water or even diet drinks. Fructose is the kind of sugar found in fruits.

Drink a glass of fructose-rich orange juice a half hour to one hour before a meal, the results suggest.

You'll eat fewer calories during the next meal and still feel comfortably full, indicates a Yale University researcher in *The American Journal of Clinical Nutrition* (51,3:428).

The diet drink, glucose-water and fructose-rich fruit juice all seem to work as appetite suppressants.

It's just that fructose worked better than sugar-water. And, the glucose-water worked better than drinks flavored with the low-calorie sweetener aspartame (brand names NutraSweet and Equal).

Plain water was least effective of the four.

In the fructose part of the study, overweight men ate nearly 300 fewer calories at lunch. Overweight women consumed an average of 431 fewer mid-day calories.

Their intakes were compared with similarly overweight men and women who drank plain water before lunch.

Even when the participants switched drinks, the results were the same. The new ones drinking the fructose-sweetened lemonade mixture ate fewer calories than those drinking the other lemonade-flavored mixtures.

But what about the calories in the fructose drink itself? You might well ask.

Since the fructose drink was about 200 calories, the net calorie suppression was about 100 to 230 calories per meal.

That still puts the orange juice diet ahead of its glucose, aspartame and plain water competition.

If only for one meal, that still adds up to a savings of 700 calories a week or 36,400 calories a year, certainly enough to make a difference over the long run.

Long-term, slow weight loss is the healthiest form of weight loss for most people.

The diet benefit, however, doesn't carry over to soft drinks sweetened with high-fructose corn syrup. People who drank a lot of aspartame-sweetened diet drinks reduced their intake of calories from sugar more than those who gulped regular soda pop, says a report three months later in the same *Journal* (51,6:963).

Maybe you are carrying around an extra 10 pounds that

keep your clothes from fitting just right. Or maybe an extra 20 or 30 pounds have accumulated over the years.

The point is, you want to be rid of the extra weight — permanently. First, the good news. You *can* lose weight, even if other diets have failed.

What's more, you don't have to starve yourself. In fact, popular sudden-weight-loss diets can cause you far more harm than good.

Even worse, crash diets might eventually make it even more difficult for you to lose weight.

However, before starting any diet, even a moderate reduction diet, check with your doctor for his okay.

Some people such as pregnant women or people with certain diseases shouldn't try to lose weight.

Caution on the 'grapefruit diet'

It took three months of vitamin and mineral treatment to pull a 47-year-old New York woman out of a diet-caused nose dive into anemia, fatigue, leg swelling and abdominal pains and bloating.

She had used the so-called grapefruit diet for two years and had lost about 50 pounds, but her health had faded during the process, according to a doctor's report in *The Journal of the American Board of Family Practice* (2,2:130). She had been eating unrestricted breakfasts, dinners and snacks but nothing at lunch but a grapefruit.

Her doctor found that she suffered from an iron deficiency, causing anemia, and a severe case of vitamin B12 shortage. The doctor put the woman in the hospital and gave her a red cell transfusion to beef up her blood. For the next three months, the doctor put the woman on a regular nutritional scheme with the addition of a multivitamin supplement, one milligram of folic acid by mouth daily, iron sulfate by mouth twice a day, and monthly injections of B12.

A year later, the woman was still eating balanced normal nutritious meals, had regained her energy and had kept her weight to within five pounds of what she weighed when she first saw the doctor, the report said. What she discarded, the doctor said, was the grapefruit diet.

The hazards of crash dieting

The sad fact is that the super-reduced-calorie diets — despite all their miracle claims — could set you up for a disaster, especially if you fall into a cycle of repeatedly gaining and losing weight.

In a Swedish study involving animals, Dr. Per Bjorntorp demonstrated that a body actually can become more efficient in gaining weight.

In other words, because of yo-yo dieting, the body might become super-efficient in turning calories into extra, unwanted weight. If that happens, you could gain more weight even if you eat less food and fewer calories.

That means you are less likely to keep weight off, and the next diet might prove to be more difficult.

Crash dieting or yo-yo dieting might also create serious

health problems.

There is the possibility that the repeated weight-loss-and-gain cycle typical of a crash-dieter could encourage heart trouble or even a stroke. This has been suggested for two reasons.

First, yo-yo dieting tends to shift weight from the hips and thighs to the stomach. According to researchers at Boston University, a heavy midsection is linked to an increased risk of stroke in men and a high rate of heart failure in both men and women.

A second concern about quick weight loss and gain is the sheer stress this kind of dieting places on the body. This strain increases the risk of sudden death from heart disease.

If near-starvation is your idea of going on a diet, it is time to change your mind.

CHAPTER 40

Yogurt and You

Remember when only dieters ate yogurt?

The many brands of yogurt on the supermarket shelves and the frozen yogurt stores popping up across the country are signs that times — and tastes — have changed. Yogurt is in.

This sudden popularity of yogurt is more than a fad.

It's based on years of medical research that suggests that for many people, fermented milk products like yogurt can help keep them in good health.

Yogurt is a good source of calcium, especially for people who have trouble digesting lactose (a milk sugar) and thus cannot drink milk.

Yogurt contains less lactose than milk, which makes it easier to digest.

Easily digestible calcium is important in preventing osteoporosis, a bone loss disease that afflicts some middle-aged and elderly women.

Fermented milk products are beneficial in treating other

conditions, too, says a report in *The American Journal of Clinical Nutrition* (49,4:675).

Indigestion, high levels of cholesterol in the blood, bowel irregularity, high blood pressure and even food poisoning have been known to yield to a diet that includes fermented milk.

Although researchers don't know the exact reasons for the benefits, they speculate that the bacteria used in fermenting milk changes the bacteria already inside the stomach and intestines.

Those changes may help the body absorb nutrients and produce enzymes needed for proper digestion of milk proteins, among other functions.

Fermented milk is identified by the bacteria it contains, and not all types are equally beneficial.

Thermophilus milk, for example, is effective in reducing lactose intolerance, but buttermilk is not.

Acidophilus milk has laxative effects in older patients. It also has slowed the growth of tumors in mice. Other studies have shown that it eliminated some forms of digestive-tract infections.

Drinking fermented milk also helps to ease travelers' diarrhea.

Yogurt bacteria, injected directly into mouse tumors, made the growths shrink, the report says.

Researchers believe that the bacteria stimulate the immune system into action, because the animals tested survived more than one bout with cancer.

Yogurt—probably the most popular form of fermented milk—also is a good source of protein, riboflavin (vitamin

B2) and folic acid (one of the B-vitamin group).

A four-ounce serving has 115 calories, about one-half that of premium ice cream, and contains a teaspoon of fat. "Light" yogurt has fewer calories and less fat.

Frozen yogurt has about the same amount of sugar, calcium, calories and protein as the equivalent amount of ice milk, but less fat.

There are some women who might raise their cancer risk by eating yogurt or other dairy products. Read about that in the Cancer chapter.

But for most folks, fermented milk like yogurt might be a good, natural way to raise overall immunity levels and fight some kinds of digestive problems.

The power of prayer: concluding remarks

The secrets in this book are based on medical reports of natural healing, but don't overlook the <u>supernatural</u> healing power of God. God is our Creator and Master Physician. If you put your faith and trust in God, by following Jesus Christ, we believe that your prayers for healing will be answered according to God's will.

Although God may not answer "yes" to every request, there is ample evidence of the power of prayer that is submissive to God's will.

Not only are there many anecdotal reports of unexplained miracles, but one scientific study has shown that prayers to "the Judeo-Christian God" were effective in treating seriously ill hospital patients.

If you would like to know more about how to know God and have eternal life through a personal relationship with Jesus Christ, please write to FC&A, Dept. JC 90, 103 Clover Green, Peachtree City, Georgia, 30269. We believe getting to know God better will change your life!